# Praise for *Hormonious*

"Navigating healthcare today can be overwhelming and leave you feeling lost. *Hormonious* provides a common sense way out by putting health back into your hands."

—James Maskell, founder of Evolution of Medicine, author of *The Community Cure*

"*Hormonious* is a beautifully crafted guide for individuals looking to reset their mind and body. With the shifts in our society, many are feeling imbalanced, stressed, and unwell. Shoshana has organized the book in a way that helps readers understand how the system became misaligned and take action to realign mind and body and achieve a youthful, healthy self. I will recommend this book to many!"

—Dr. Trupti Gokani, board certified neurologist and ayurvedic wellness coach, author of *The Mysterious Mind*

"When medicine becomes super specialized—and we do have specialties for the right ear versus the left one—we still need specialties to encompass the body as one unit. *Hormonious* by Karen Bernstein Shoshana tries to fulfill this mission. This book is worth a read by anyone suffering from perplexing chronic symptoms."

—Dr. Yehuda Shoenfeld, professor emeritus, founder and head of Zabludowicz Center for Autoimmune Diseases, Sheba Medical Center

"If you're looking for insight into what's behind your 'hormonal' symptoms, this book is the place to start! In *Hormonious*, Karen Shoshana walks us through the different processes of the body, what dysfunction may look like, and how to approach our symptoms through a functional nutrition lens."

—Andrea Nakayama, functional medicine nutritionist,
founder of Functional Nutrition Alliance

"*Hormonious* provides a functional medicine overview for women, revealing the serious harms of processed foods and chronic stress and addressing the inevitable impact of menopause and the transitional years. This book can greatly help women move beyond bad habits and embrace a functional approach to wellness."

—Dr. Felice Gersh, integrative gynecologist,
author of *PCOS SOS*

# Hormonious

## THE FUNCTIONAL APPROACH TO OPTIMAL WELLNESS, BOUNDLESS ENERGY & GLOWING LONGEVITY

## Karen Bernstein Shoshana
Functional Diagnostic Nutrition Practitioner
Certified Holistic Health Coach

wellness girl
PUBLISHING

*I dedicate this book to every woman who is suffering from her symptoms  and who also struggles to get the answers to her health issues. You are my inspiration because I was you.*

*And, for my mother, whose beautiful life has always been a model for mine and whose tragic health descent helped to galvanize my purpose.*

# TABLE OF CONTENTS

# PREFACE

The day my mom made and tried to serve multiple pieces of burnt toast and then used salt in place of sugar in her famous butter cookies, my life changed. I knew right then that something was very wrong, but it took a number of months and frequent cajoling of both my parents to make an appointment with the family doctor as well as a neurologist. My dad was in denial too. Once she went and we received the sad news of her diagnosis, we all felt the blow. My beautiful, loving, educated mother—a talented baker, skilled tennis player, avid reader, former bacteriologist, and Holocaust survivor— had joined the ranks of those suffering from Alzheimer's disease.

Watching her body and brain deteriorate and her memory of me slowly blur was not just a harrowing experience. It redefined me to myself. Who are you when your mother doesn't remember you? I had to rethink who I was and, of course, I could not help but seriously consider whether I might face the same fate.

My mother generally ate well and was social, active, engaged— all the things they say are helpful in preventing this terrible, heart-breaking disease. She was an apparently normal, healthy 76-year-old woman with a properly functioning body, or so it seemed. Aside from the memory slips, there were no other symptoms any of us detected. There was no other cause for alarm, nothing else giving my mom or her family a "head's up" about what was brewing in her brain or that it had been deteriorating for years. At least nothing that we could associate with a decline in her memory. I asked myself again and again: How could this have happened?

Could we have prevented it?

How could I help save others from my mother's fate?

What if this happens to me?

My path to helping myself and others was inspired by my mom and the tragic turn her life took. Illnesses and problems with the body often show symptoms long before they turn into a life-threatening situation. I wanted to learn which lifestyle choices and factors made a difference in fighting off chronic disease. Maybe there were signs but we had missed them.

You are reading *Hormonious* for a reason. It may be that you are already wondering whether (or already know that) chronic disease—maybe Alzheimer's, autoimmunity, cancer, heart disease, or any number of other health issues—could be in your future. Are you on that slippery slope? If you are already experiencing chronic symptoms of stress, fatigue, and sleeplessness, the answer may be yes, but this is just the tip of the iceberg. There are hundreds of other signs that you are on a path to declining health. Is your digestion off? Do you have skin issues, headaches, irritability, mood swings, or food sensitivities? Joint or body pain? Brain fog? Is your memory becoming unreliable? Are loved ones and friends pointing this out to you? One or more of these indicators may be signs that your health is not what it could be, and that you may be headed in the wrong direction.

If you have sought outside help for your vague and troublesome symptoms, chances are that the medical guidance you have received has only focused on treating those problems directly. Unfortunately, masking your body's manifestations of dysfunction does nothing to change the inward conditions that are triggering them and causing the dysfunction in the first place.

But guess what? There is another way. There is a method for wellness that looks at you—not just your symptoms, but the *whole you*—as someone who is different from anyone else. There is a way of seeing your life through a lens that can help you discover what you are doing to create disease, and what you could do to create health, from the inside out. Hormones are the key to the equation of what makes you *you*. They are the ultimate personalized internal response to life, and the more you get to know them and learn to manipulate them, the more easily you will be able to regain and maintain optimal health. If you're ready to get serious, arm yourself with the steps to regain control, and set yourself on a journey towards true healing and ultimate wellness, I can help you start at the beginning.

The beginning of a truly Hormonious *you*.

## WHAT'S IN IT FOR YOU?

Nobody cares as much about your health as you do. Not even your doctor. And nobody can make the changes good health demands except *you*.

But first, you need to know how. My aim is to provide a framework of health for you to follow, and a step-by-step plan to orient you and get you moving towards your health goals. Health isn't simply about one thing—it's not just about gluten, or fat, or grains, or sugar. It's not about going keto, paleo or vegan. It's not about that one food that gives you a stomachache or the latest hot supplement or herb. It's not just about exercise, or meditation, or stress management. But it can be about all of those things, and more.

Health encompasses a much wider scope than any one philosophy or practice. It includes everything that is happening inside *and outside* the body. Your history, your genetics, your physiology, your choices, and your body's interaction with its environment are all at play. Your hormones play a central role, one that influences your health and the troubling symptoms you're wrangling with in uncountable ways. Understanding what triggers their over- or underproduction means that you can have an important role in their management. In this book, we will journey together towards the interior of you, and then we will journey outward again, to examine and recalibrate all the facets of your life that constitute your health and that are critical to your "big picture." It's going to be an exciting journey—one that will connect with and rely on your internal compass (that voice that calls your attention to your pain, where it comes from, and what you should be doing about it).

# INTRODUCTION

## What Is Health?

The *Oxford English Dictionary* defines health as: "The state of being free from illness or injury." On the face of it, if you are not injured or sick right now, you're healthy. But there is another definition. The second definition Oxford offers is: "A person's physical or mental condition." This one resonates more deeply with me and what I practice. Health is not just the absence of sickness. It is a direct reflection of someone's condition. It is how they present to the world, and how they feel inside. A perfect example of this is someone experiencing chronic stress. Are they ill or injured? Of course not. However, that doesn't mean they are healthy.

In fact, they are not. At least, they are not in optimal health.

Optimal health is a state of fine balance and requires a perfect interplay between genetics, environment, and physiology. To achieve it is the work of a lifetime, and that is something bigger than what I can share with you in this book. This is just a beginning—a primer on health. My wish for you is that you can learn and begin to enact the steps necessary to get you to a place where you feel fabulous and then your life can just keep getting better.

I want this for you because I know how "crappy" feels, and I also know how "amazing" feels. I believe each one of us is entitled to feel amazing in this life, and I know this is attainable. It's not necessarily constant or perpetually sustainable, because life is unpredictable and, invariably, things go wrong—they break, we trip, we fall. Big life events, good and bad, are going to happen to you. Disease and death are realities, and the current state of the world, including the environment, is enough to send anyone into a tailspin. And certainly the unfolding of COVID-19 has impacted you and added its own layer of stressors. Life will inevitably feel overwhelming, but that's all part of the dance. To get through it you need to build a resilient backbone of health. After all, you only have this one life, and a glass half empty still has water in it to drink.

I also want to mention another caveat. If you are in a rush to get healthy immediately, the content of this book may be hard for you to hear. Health is complex, and when it has gone far out of balance, it will take time to restore it. However, although building a strong foundation of health takes time, fortunately you have tools to turn things around, right here, at your disposal. Take a deep breath in. Hold it, then let it out.

Do that one more time. Inhale...hold... and a slow exhale out.

Okay, let's get started.

## Elevate the Patient in the Patient-Doctor Relationship

Today, physicians are crunched for time and can't necessarily delve deeply into your particulars—certainly not in one office visit or zoom call. They also may not be on top of current studies and research, which are critical to understanding health today. Certainly, they are not trained in nutrition or to look at the big picture of lifestyle as it impacts all aspects of health and wellness (though that is changing somewhat, thankfully).

Rather, physicians learn to assign a drug to relieve a symptom or diagnose a condition that has reached the disease state. They don't consider the wide expanse between health and disease, where vague or seemingly inexplicable symptoms lie, but this is just where a functional medicine approach could provide a different perspective. Pharmaceutical companies have certainly played a big part in this. They are motivated to profit by the sale of medications they have developed, and while some medications can be lifesaving, necessary, and useful for relieving acute conditions, many are simply bandages that cover problems but do not resolve them. A slew of commercials bombard us every day, encouraging us to ask for these medications, even though they are not fixing our problems and are causing even worse side effects.

I am not dissing doctors. My dad was one and my brother is one, too. I respect and appreciate the field immensely. But we have to tame our expectations of and elevate our standing in the patient-doctor relationship by participating as equal partners. I believe this is the only way to get to the bottom of any chronic health issue. It's time for every patient and potential patient to ask themselves: *Who do you trust? How do you know what's true?* We are all overwhelmed by the wave of health information now available to anyone with a computer or a smartphone, and most of us have already recognized how much of that information is confusing, blatantly contradictory, misleading, or even completely wrong. It's frustrating and unhelpful in the quest for wellness.

## Wellness Begins with Education

I wrote this book for every woman who wants more—not only to regain control of her health, but also to learn how her body functions so that she can become her own best advocate and the heroine in her own health journey. This book comes out of a long search to discover not just what bodies need, but why so many women are suffering.

During my training in functional nutrition and integrative health, I learned a lot of exciting and applicable information that set me on my path to help women heal and thrive, but at every stage of my education journey, I felt I could still learn more. When I began to take on clients, I recognized that I was seeing some of the same issues over and over—common symptoms such as chronic stress, fatigue, inability to sleep through the night, brain fog, and mood swings. Weight that won't budge continues to be a typical complaint. These common symptoms cropped up in a wide variety of people, many of whom seemed to be living healthy lives. This made me question what we all consider to be "healthy living." When I looked closer, I realized that most of my clients:

- Thought they were eating right, but weren't.

- Were exercising, but often in a way that was actually adding stress, rather than reducing it.

- Knew sleep was important but still couldn't seem to get enough, and didn't understand why.

- Did not recognize how overwhelmed and stressed they were on a daily basis, and were therefore not actively managing that stress.

- Thought they were doing a good job and in general, didn't think they really had to change that much (and didn't want to).

- Wanted me to help them resolve "just a few little problems," apparently not seeing the bigger picture of how their every act influenced their health.

Where was the disconnect between true health and these misguided perceptions? The more I worked with clients, the more I recognized two things I wanted to be able to do:

- First, I wanted the road to healing to be more efficient. I wanted this for myself firstly, but I also wanted to offer this to my clients. Why waste time with 10 steps when you could get there in two?

- Second, I wanted to have a deeper knowledge of the science behind chronic health issues common to women. I felt compelled to dig more deeply into the biochemical mechanisms behind health dysfunctions, to help my clients heal.

Through my studies in Functional Diagnostic Nutrition, the disparate elements finally came together. I learned more about how food can be used as medicine to address and improve or resolve many chronic health issues and their symptoms. I learned how lab testing can identify malfunctions and uncover healing opportunities—saving time, money, and frustration. I learned what was going on "behind the scenes" of vague symptoms and, especially, how hormones exerted their profound influence on the workings of a woman's body. Seeing how the interior was functioning made all the difference. Clients could finally begin to understand exactly what was happening inside them and why, and as a result were even more motivated to make changes. Lab test results that gave credence to symptoms were both valuable and validating for them.

Bringing all these tools together for my clients—especially education about how their own bodies worked and the accountability that comes from having a health coach, as well as access to tests that could help them pinpoint where things were going wrong—created a new and more powerful spirit of change in my practice. My clients found the science of health more accessible and the steps to health more manageable. They were able to see and feel progress without feeling overwhelmed. They began to understand the connection between what they ate and how they felt, and to feel the benefits of incorporating breathing exercises and other stress management techniques into their lives. Over time, I watched each of them experience their own epiphanies as they finally comprehended that their health was a direct product of their effort, their interest, and, ultimately, their responsibility. They recognized that nobody cared as much about their health as they did, and nobody else could make the changes that good health demands but themselves.

I finally felt like I was genuinely helping people in a profound way. My next step was to help *more people*. Since I can only take on so many clients, I decided to write this book so that I could deliver this message to a broader audience, helping more women take those same actions and have those same realizations. This book is designed to hold that space for you. I'll tell you stories about women who probably share many of your symptoms and experiences (myself included), and I'll explain the science of what might be going wrong for you in simple terms. I've created several (downloadable) worksheets to support your efforts, and I'll describe them later in the book.

I know that you are here because in some way, or in several ways, you are hurting. Maybe you feel that you are floating in a sea of information and it's overwhelming, or you aren't sure what to believe. I've got you. I am here to help you because (and I want you to believe this because it's true): you deserve to feel good. You deserve to be healthy so you can make the most of your life. This world is better when women are healthy, confident, and strong. And the world needs us now more than ever. So, let's do this!

## HOW TO USE THIS BOOK

I've laid this book out to be read from beginning to end. A good portion of Chapter 1 is an in-depth prompting of your health history—feel free to browse and return as you begin to fill in the pieces of your own health document. Generally, you can jump around, but if you really want to get organized with your health, start where all health begins: in the gut – this is Chapter 2. It took me many years to appreciate the link between the gut and overall health, but once you learn the relationship between your digestive system and the rest of your body, you will be more attuned to the power of the choices you make.

Our bodies are complex systems of organs, tissues, communication networks, and interdependent moving parts. We even have a built-in defense structure—our immune system—to protect us. Did you know that your skin, your largest organ, is the first line of that defense? Because of this amazing interconnectivity, you will probably notice that concepts raised in one chapter of this book will relate to and intertwine with those in other chapters. Chapters are segregated by common, big-picture symptoms that are related to underlying hormones and systems, and I'll expand on those as we go. You'll also note common themes throughout that will be tied up for you neatly in the end, but just remember that every part of your body impacts every other part in some way. As you will soon learn, this is one of the foundational elements of functional medicine. When you see advice repeated, it isn't because I am being unoriginal! It is because some practices effectively address problems in multiple areas.

My goal is to help you learn, apply, and correct for whole-body health. To understand the inner workings, we need to narrow in and focus on different areas with specificity, while at the same time, stand back for perspective and understand that as we are investigating for an underlying cause or causes to correct an imbalance, we are also aiming to treat the whole body.

If you take this step by step, and integrate the lessons I provide in Hormonious, you will be making changes that will serve you for the rest of your life. Your particular symptoms will determine which Fix Its from each chapter make sense for you. Just remember, achieving good health does not happen overnight. Your health dysfunction and the development of your symptoms didn't happen overnight, either. But with the consistent practice of good health habits you will learn in this book, you can get there, maybe even faster than you think. As I mentioned above, I've developed several worksheets to support you in this process to keep you organized, accountable, and successful. You can download them at wellnessgirl.net/hormoniousplan—you'll learn more about them in Chapter 7. Use them to achieve the health you desire. We'll do it together. We're going to get you to shine. We're going to make you Hormonious.

# CHAPTER 1

# PACKING FOR YOUR TRIP TO HEALTH

*"Be ruthless for your own well-being."*
*—Holly Butcher*

Your wellness is the single most important factor in living a rich and rewarding life, and it is *the reason* I wrote this book. But wellness is complex, influenced by a multitude of factors, many of which are happening inside your body right now. You have more control over those factors than you may realize. Your digestion, your microbiome, your dietary choices, your lifestyle choices, your *chronic stress* (that's a big one), and the whole dance of your hormones—each has a part to play. The better you understand how it all works and how what you do directly influences all these factors, the sooner you can capture that elusive-seeming state of optimal health.

To get there, let's work together. I have information for you, and my hope is that you can begin to notice and hone in on your symptoms, keep track of them, and make the changes that work for you. To move in a different direction, you must do different things. This is essential to the process. So is the recognition that everything happening around you and to you either becomes a part of your journey towards wellness, or a part of your journey away from it.

This is a significant piece of the puzzle, and you will soon understand why. Later in this chapter, I will introduce you to the concept of the functional timeline, and the Functional Timeline Plus that you will be filling out to keep track of your own health story. This document will become the centerpiece and guiding star on your mission to sound health. It is the place where you will record all the pieces of the puzzle that is you.

To illustrate this point more precisely, I'd like to start by telling you my story. I hope this will get you thinking more about *your* story so that you can start to reflect on your own life and its major events, both good and bad.

## My Path from Patient to Practitioner

When my mother developed Alzheimer's disease, I knew the whole family had a difficult road ahead, but what I didn't know at the time was that the year following my mom's death would be an especially challenging one for me. I'd thought about my parents' death from an early age. While they didn't speak much of their traumatic childhoods (my dad was a Holocaust survivor too), I had a deep understanding, an intuitive feeling, that their survival, and ultimately my existence, was a matter of perfect chance. Their complete and utter devotion to me and my two older brothers was a combination of genuine love and a desire to distance themselves from their past. We were the physical testimony of their survival. And as the youngest and only daughter, I had reserved extra space in my heart to oversee my parents' care and their decline. I considered it my honor and believed that their passage into old age and death deserved the utmost care, respect, and reverence—not only because they were my parents, but because of the generous, kind souls they each were. I felt blessed.

My mom's last year was heart-wrenching to watch. At the time she passed, I felt relief. I believed she did, too. The long agony of watching her decline was over, and in the months following her death, I sincerely thought I was fine. What I didn't realize was that a crisis was brewing within me and was preparing to erupt. Several months later, it did.

At first, I noticed something was off in my body, but I couldn't put my finger on it. I wrote it off as hormones. I was in my mid-40s and expected the normal decline of female hormones that happens during perimenopause as the body prepares to turn off the procreation tap. If you had asked me what I was feeling then, I would have had a difficult time putting it into words. It was a new feeling, that much I knew. I was tired, sure. No energy, yup. I was not my usual perky self. But on top of all that, there was an actual, strange, and unusual sensation running through my body that I didn't recognize. It was like a pulse or vibration and I didn't like it. It felt at odds with how I normally felt. Something wasn't right.

So I did the usual. I ignored it. Until it began to feel more urgent. I visited my gynecologist, since I thought it was hormonal. When that didn't result in any information, I visited my family doctor. Everything looked normal. I even went the extra step of visiting a holistic doctor. Not only did nothing show up in my general lab results, but I was told that there was nothing wrong and that I should return to my life, the bottom line being that there was no relief they could offer me. Unless something was showing up on a conventional lab test, or there was a diagnosable disorder, nothing could be done.

This was all extremely frustrating. I knew that something was going on, but no medical expert was able to help me. And though my description of this strange sensation did not provide any insights, the holistic doctor (in an effort, I suspect, to provide me with something that would at least *seem* like a remedy for my symptoms) gave me a hormone cream that in only one day turned me into an emotional wreck. Not the answer I needed. Massages, acupuncture, and Chinese medicine didn't help, either. Neither did herbal supplements, essential oils, sound baths, focused breathing, visualization, or meditation. Hypnosis actually provided a semblance of relief, though not enough to get me out of a downward-spiraling cycle.

So, yes, I tried it all! What was left? I felt I had nowhere to turn. In desperation, I decided to focus on the only thing that I felt I had control over: despite how I felt, I needed to figure out what I was going to do for the rest of my life. I was a woman at a crossroads, standing alone in the large vacuum that my mother had left. I'm not sure whether I realized at the time that it was my mom's death that prompted me to feel like I needed to make a complete and total re-evaluation of myself, but in retrospect, that was certainly the reason. The death of a loved one can be transformative, but at the time, I only felt that if I couldn't nail down a solution to my symptoms, at least I could be actively engaged in my quest to find my life purpose. If there was no answer to my health problems, I would try to move past them and live my life. I was determined to make a plan of action.

## The Gift of Functional Medicine

But what would this action be? I looked back over my life and recognized that I had always been fascinated by health and had spent most of my life reading and thinking about it. Now, as a victim of my own health crisis and a witness to my mother's tragic disease, I realized that maybe this was my path and had been all along. I decided to pursue this field with purpose and determination.

First, I studied at the Institute for Integrative Nutrition, and became a health coach. That was gratifying and I loved my work, but I also felt compelled to have a better understanding of the science behind my advice and guidance. I wanted to learn precisely what was happening on the inside of the body. What were the organs and systems at play in both dysfunction and in health? Functional Nutrition Alliance (formerly Holistic Nutrition Lab) was my next step and where I began my advanced training. With that context and knowledge, I was able to inspire a deeper commitment from my clients. The more I learned, the more they did, too, which meant the dedication to their health was stronger.

I first learned about functional medicine while I was studying at IIN. Dr. Mark Hyman, physician, author, and IFM Board President of Clinical Affairs, was a presenter, and I was immediately taken with the premise. The functional medicine model "evolved from the insights and perspectives of a small group of influential thought leaders who realized the importance of an individualized approach to disease causes based on the evolving research in nutritional science, genomics, and epigenetics."[1] Wow! Functional medicine is essentially the smarter, sexier, and also the more practical (and practicable) version of conventional medicine. It focuses on mechanisms and causes rather than just symptoms and diseases, and prioritizes lifestyle and dietary therapies (things anyone can choose to do) over pharmaceutical medicine. That made a lot of sense to me. It sounded like the medicine of the future!

To put it in simple terms, functional medicine (I'll call it FM from now on) determines how and why illness occurs and uses a systems-based approach to restore health by addressing the root causes of disease for each individual. It values the therapeutic relationship with the patient and considers not only the symptoms and organs at issue, but how every system of the body contributes to or fights against health dysfunction. It also takes the old saying to heart, that "all disease begins in the gut," by focusing on the primacy of the digestive system. This is common-sense medicine.

At its core, FM believes that nutrition and the health of the digestive tract are key components to wellness. For example, if you are experiencing a chronic skin eruption of some sort, a conventional approach would be to go to a dermatologist. That doctor might prescribe a cream to calm the irritation. An FM doctor would take a completely different approach, considering your diet, your environment, and stressors that you've been experiencing, in an attempt to discover the origin of the rash. After taking an in-depth health history, that FM doctor may recommend additions and/or subtractions to your diet along with lifestyle tweaks. After assessing your serum labs from your annual check-up, additional functional lab tests may be in order. Putting ointment on the infected area might turn out to be one mode of treatment, but the FM approach takes into account that skin eruptions have causes that are literally more than skin deep. Do you have an allergy? To what, and why? Or maybe your liver is overloaded, or your immune system is attacking your skin. Perhaps you were exposed to a toxin, or had an adverse reaction to something you ate. Each of these causes would have different treatments, even to similarly appearing rashes. You can probably see why this is a much more thorough and effective approach to a seemingly simple problem and why a cream alone may temporarily calm a rash, but probably doesn't cure it.

I responded deeply to this philosophy of health and learned everything I could about it because it made so much sense to me. It has become my approach to every health problem I see in my clients, as well as in myself, because it is the most effective way I have discovered to understand where health begins and how anyone can achieve it for themselves.

As you'll notice in the questions posed by the Functional Timeline Plus, FM also elevates the importance of lifestyle. While the word "lifestyle" may seem like a buzzword, to me it is timeless and comprehensive. It includes not just your diet and exercise but all facets of your life from relationships, parenting, and career to sleep, stress, and your environment. FM offers a way to address your health challenges through the lens of your lifestyle. I sometimes wonder how my health would have evolved if I'd had access to FM during my own tumultuous time.

Here's something else to remember—and you'll hear me say this throughout: *Symptoms of sub-optimal health are common, but that does not mean they are normal.* This, or some version of this, is practically an FM mantra. Keep that in mind throughout this process and beyond. This is my invitation to you to stop ignoring or merely suppressing the symptoms you may experience. *They mean something.* Symptoms are a message from your body that something isn't right. Acknowledge and keep track of them (I'm going to show you how) like they are clues to a great mystery. Because that is exactly what they are: clues to the mystery of *you.*

> FUNCTIONAL MEDICINE states on its website: "[E]ach symptom or differential diagnosis may be one of many contributing to an individual's illness..., [and] functional medicine treatment targets the specific manifestations of disease in each individual." The site goes on to explain that a single cause may result in a different diagnosis in different people. For example, inflammation may cause depression in one person, but can be the cause of heart disease, cancer, arthritis, or diabetes in someone else. Similarly, depression may be caused by inflammation in one person, but have a different cause in another, such as a Vitamin D deficiency, low thyroid levels, antibiotic use,[2] or stressful life events. Because we are all different and will have differing root causes, a different protocol will be required for each person. Thus, we need a comprehensive document that will reflect our individual health experiences so that we can refer back to it when needed.

What I am going to ask you to do next is to engage in a reckoning of your entire health history, from before you were born to this present moment. I do not ask this of you cavalierly. This is the beginning of a journey towards health that could completely transform the way you treat yourself. It is deeply meaningful and crucial for the work we will be doing together. Because you are reading this book, I assume that there is something in your life you want to change, so please consider every question and answer it as fully as you can. Let's find out the exact nature of what that is.

## THE FUNCTIONAL TIMELINE PLUS

If you were my client coming to see me, one of the first things I would do is a functional timeline of your health. This is a cool tool FM uses to help collect, categorize, and organize chronic symptoms.

Remember, FM's primary objective (and mine...and now yours!) is to seek out the reasons for why you are not feeling your best. We aren't patching symptoms. We are transforming bodies!

Figuring this out requires some detective work--the more you dig, the more you'll see the connections between your health challenges and the road that brought you here. The functional timeline will help you organize the chronology of your life. It will be your road map and first step in taking a stand for your health. You may even notice feeling emotional or experiencing some catharsis (relief and understanding) during this process as you finally put to paper what's happening for you right now, and what has been happening to you throughout your entire life leading up to this moment.

Please take a look at Table 1 to see the sample used by FM practitioners. In Table 2, I've provided you with a sample of the version I have created especially for you. It both enhances and simplifies the timeline used by FM physicians, so I'll refer to it as the Functional Timeline Plus or FTP throughout the book. You can find the complete FTP to download at wellnessgirl.net/hormoniousplan. Have a look at the example and then read on to do your own. You could write your answers on a printed-out form, or keep them in a file on your computer. However you do it, have it easily available so you can always add to it as necessary and take it to your doctor's appointments.

# Table 1:

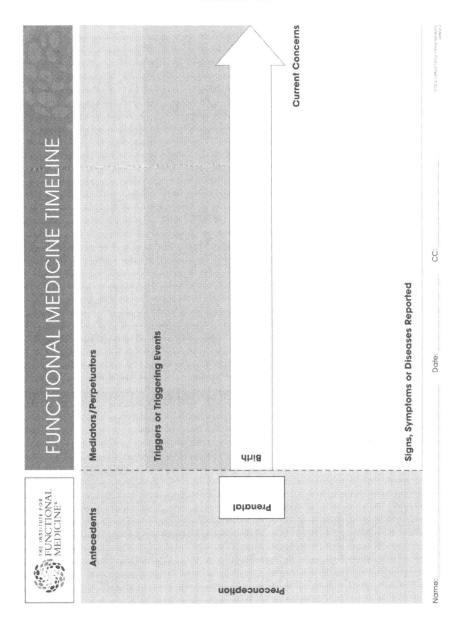

# Table 2:

HORMONIOUS

## FUNCTIONAL
## TIMELINE PLUS

Name: _____

Date: _____

| ANTECEDENTS (GENETICS, FAMILY HISTORY) | MEDIATORS (YOUR ACTIONS, THOUGHTS, CIRCUMSTANCES, ETC.) | TRIGGERS (FOOD SENSITIVITIES, STRESSORS, TOXIN EXPOSURE, ETC.) |
|---|---|---|

PRENATAL/PRECONCEPTION

Birth:

Birth to now:

SIGNS, SYMPTOMS OR DISEASE(S)

Current concerns:

Lab tests:                                     Medications/Supplements:

Download a blank version at wellnessgirl.net/hormoniousplan

# Prenatal and Preconception

First let's fill out the section about you *before* you were born. Yep, that's when it all started for you. Your first consideration is the health of your mom while she was pregnant with you, and even before she got pregnant with you. If it's possible to have a conversation with your mom about this, now is the time to ask these questions. (If you are not able to ask her, think about whether anyone else would know the answers, or fill them in to the best of your knowledge. It's okay if you don't know the answer to every question.) Research shows that the health of the mother during and even prior to pregnancy can affect the health and genetic expression of her baby. You are establishing the nature of your environment even before you came into the world, which is valuable information in determining your disease risk and genetic picture, as well as other more subtle aspects of your pre-birth environment.

- How would your birth mother describe the state of her own health *before* getting pregnant? Did she have any major illnesses or other chronic problems?

- How would she describe the state of her health *during* pregnancy? Did she get sick? Was she taking any medications, such as antibiotics, anti-depressants, or medications for morning sickness or other pregnancy symptoms? Did she have any diagnosed problems like gestational diabetes or pre-eclampsia?

- Did she think she had an easy pregnancy? Or was it difficult? If difficult, what did she feel was difficult about it?

- What was her life like at that time? Was pregnancy a time of love and excitement for her, or was it stressful? Did she have a lot of family support, or not so much?

- Did either of your parents experience any trauma in their lives? (Studies[3, 4, 5] show that childhood trauma alters genes that can be passed onto future generations.)

## Antecedents

Antecedents are factors, genetic or acquired, that you brought with you into the world that may predispose you to illness. These include family history, genetics, and the circumstances of your birth and delivery. The more information you have, the better. For example, if there is a family history of GI disorders or depression or autoimmunity, that would go here. If you can get some basic genetic testing, put any relevant results here. Taking the time to do this is worthwhile because you will have this information recorded all in one place—it can be easy to forget things when you need to know them, such as at a doctor's visit. Also, it will help you to have these things in the forefront of your mind, for motivational purposes, as you pursue your health goals. Finally, discovering that you may have a condition in common with a relative can be validating and instructive. How are they handling it? What are they doing to address it? Family members can be another resource on your road of learning.

- What is your family history as it relates to illness and disease?

  o Did your parents or grandparents (and so on) have diagnosed diseases? List those here.

- Do you know if you carry any gene mutation that could increase your risk of getting any diseases such as cancer, Alzheimer's disease, Parkinson's, or autoimmunity? Having a genetic mutation does not mean that a disease state will express itself. But knowing your genetic propensities can help you assess your diet and lifestyle, take preventive steps, and upgrade your health practices to give yourself the best opportunity to keep that gene turned off.

- Were there any particular circumstances surrounding your birth that were atypical? Mention that briefly here, as you'll be describing your birth in more detail later.

## Mediators/Perpetuators

Mediators are the things you are doing, the conditions you are living in, and even the thoughts and emotions you are having in your life currently, that are perpetuating, rather than changing, your current health condition. They can be either positive or negative, and could be making your circumstances either better or worse. Examples of positive mediators are eating a balanced diet, meditating, exercising, and traveling to see the world or having other interesting experiences. These are activities that are known to enhance health. Examples of negative mediators are insufficient sleep, chronic stress, eating foods that you are sensitive or reactive to, or being largely sedentary. (On the other hand, for someone who is in a state of adrenal exhaustion, vigorous exercise would be an example of a negative mediator.) Being in a toxic relationship is also considered a mediator. Although you may not know everything you are doing that could be causing health issues for you right now, make your best guess. Here are some cues, but if you think of other mediators relevant to you, add those, then circle the positive ones and put an X by the negatives.

- Do you eat a lot of refined or packaged foods? How often?
- Do you eat a lot of fiber-containing carbs, such as vegetables and minimally processed whole grains? How often?
- Do you drink alcohol? How much?
- Do you eat a lot of sugary foods? How often?

- Do you eat a lot of fried foods? How often?

- Do you have any ongoing hormone-related issues?

- Do you have any ongoing immune-related issues?

- Are you experiencing any ongoing psychological stress?

- Are you experiencing any ongoing exposure to environmental insults, such as mold or chemicals?

- Describe your sleep. Do you go to sleep late? Is it difficult to fall asleep? Do you wake in the middle of the night? Are you getting at least seven hours of sleep on most nights?

- Do you exercise for at least 30 minutes on most days?

- Do you regularly participate in activities that you enjoy?

## Triggers or Triggering Events

Triggers are the things that could be provoking a negative health state, or predispose you to a higher risk of disease or chronic conditions or symptoms. Some examples of a trigger or triggering event:

- Eating the wrong diet for your needs

- Exposure to environmental toxins or antigens

- Chronic stress, injury, or trauma

- Infection with a virus or bacteria

- Medication use (such as antibiotic or steroid use)

Try to think of all the possibilities and list them.

## Birth

Here, you'll list your date of birth and describe any other accompanying details:

My date of birth:

- What was your birth weight?
- Were you born prematurely or late? By how much?
- Did you have any health problems right after birth?
- Were you born vaginally or by C-section?
- Were you breastfed or bottle fed? If you were breastfed, for how long?
- Was your hospital stay extended for any reason?

## Birth to Now

Now it's time to think back and list every single health event throughout your life, from birth until now. Include things that happened to you in childhood, teenage years, young adulthood, and so on. If you have access to earlier health records, consult them for information. This section will make up the major part of your timeline. On reflection, you may not think you should include the time that you had measles, or a UTI, but guess what? Those can influence your long-term health. If you took antibiotics for an illness, add that to the list. Keeping track of how many times you've had antibiotics over the course of your life will be eye-opening to you when you read about the digestive system and the microbiome in Chapter 2. If it was frequent, even if you have no idea how often, you will know the answer is "often," and that, too, is significant.

List the following:

- Accidents
- Allergy history (environmental and food allergies)
- Any surgery or major illness
- Births of your own children
- Bouts of severe depression
- Death of family members or close friends

- Dental history (amalgams, root canals, other surgeries)
- Exposure to trauma(s)
- Extreme travel (such as to a developing country or involving extreme physical exertion)
- Extreme work environments (such as those involving extreme physical exertion or exposure to extreme conditions)
- Major emotional upheaval
- Major injuries
- Marriage
- Separation, divorce (for yourself and/or other family members)
- Stressful or life-changing events from the moment you left the hospital after delivery
- Unusually recurrent minor illness (like constant ear infections or migraines)
- Any other major experiences or transitions, like moving, graduation, advanced education, or anything else you remember

## Current Concerns

What do you worry about in your life right now? Do you have concerns about your health, your family, your career, your friends, or anything else? If you currently suffer from a health condition, consider what life events might have happened right before the onset. List anything and everything, and corresponding dates if you know them (or make your best guess). Keep adding to the list if other concerns develop, and whenever you can, record the date that a concern began and the date it is resolved. (As you proceed with this timeline, don't delete issues that have resolved. This history will help you evaluate your own progress as you get healthier.)

List all your concerns here, including:

- When did you last feel really well and healthy?

- How long have you been experiencing symptoms that interfere with your life?

- What do you think caused or might be contributing to your current health state?

## Signs, Symptoms, or Diseases Reported

This information is for any diagnosed disease(s) or symptom(s) you are currently experiencing. To make this a living, evolving document, make sure to indicate the date associated with any signs and symptoms as well as length of time you have been experiencing them. Some things to consider:

- Do you have GI symptoms like bloating, constipation, diarrhea, heartburn, gas, or cramping after eating?

- How often do you eliminate (poop)? Indicate the frequency, quality, and ease or difficulty of passing your stools. (Ideal is at least once a day but no more than three times a day, and stool that exits your body cleanly with no residue on your bum or the bowl.)

- Do you have skin issues?

- Hair loss?

- Energy challenges?

- How is your mood?

- Are you experiencing any pain?

## Your Vision of Health

Although this timeline is based on the FM model, for our purposes I have added a couple of sections to expand the context of your health. The best way to make something happen is to take steps towards it. To that end, write out your vision of health here:

- If you could erase three problems with a magic wand, what would they be?

- What is your vision of health? How would you like your body to function in a perfect world?

- Think back to the last time you were healthy and happy. What did you have then that you don't have now?

- What will you do when you achieve optimal health that you can't do now?

- How will your life be different than it is now?

**Hormonious Tip:** Tell your future self that you are looking out for her, and that this is your plan for her life. Tell her that when she is 95 years old, she will look back with a clear head and a sincere smile, and think to herself, "I did it my way! I did everything I wanted to do, and if I didn't, I sure as hell tried my best!"

## Current Way of Eating, AKA Your Diet

When I use the word "diet," I'm not referring to any particular one, unless I clearly say so. In general, your diet is your way of eating. Use one recent week as a guideline for reference and try to be as specific as possible.

- What do you eat for breakfast?
- Lunch?

- Dinner?

- Snacks?

- Do you have dessert often?

- Do you eat out often?

- How often do you drink alcohol?

- Do you smoke? If so, how much?

- Do you engage in "extracurricular" pot-smoking? How often?

- Do you snack on sweets? How often? What kind?

- Is there a particular food that you eat more of than what you think is normal, or that you get frequent cravings for?

### Functional Nutrition Is the Gateway to Optimal Health

Functional nutrition lies at the heart of FM, as functional nutrition emphasizes the importance of high-quality foods to address imbalances in the body and "move individuals toward the highest expression of health."[6] Science is confirming that food is powerfully influential and that poor-quality food can actually create disease. Food is information, not just energy. It tells your body how to function, literally signaling the cells to behave as needed. You want those cells getting the best possible information so that your body is functioning optimally.

## Lifestyle + Your Environment

Everything about your current lifestyle other than food goes here. Think about everything that goes into or on your body: the foods you eat that contain pesticides or other chemicals, the air you breathe, the products you use on your body and in your life, your exposure to cell phones and electromagnetic fields (EMFs), and the toxins you are surrounded by. These all have a potential impact on your health. Think about these questions and record your answers:

- What's your current average level of stress?

- Do you exercise?

- How are your relationships?

- How are your friendships? Do you have a supportive group of friends? Large or small?

- How is your work life? Is it a career or just a job? Do you love it?

- How do you feel about money?

- How do you see your future?

- How would you describe your best and worst habits? What are they?

- Do you have interesting hobbies or a dedicated passion?

- How does your life feel to you right now?

- Do you practice a religion, or have a spiritual outlet?

- What is your environment like both at home and at work? Are you exposed to any chemicals[7] or mold that might be harming your health?

## Lab Tests

When was the last time you went to your doctor for a physical and to have a complete blood count (CBC) performed? If it's been a while, this is the place to start. I won't begin working with someone until they have that information within the past year, preferably within the last six months. Your doctor will probably want to check your cholesterol, A1C (an indicator of average blood sugar), and blood pressure—if not, request these. Other labs to request include your Vitamin D levels, ferritin (iron), B12 and methylmalonic acid (MMA; a better indicator of B12 utilization), C-reactive protein (CRP; inflammatory marker), homocysteine, and magnesium. These should be part and parcel of every annual physical, whether you're experiencing symptoms or not. Tracking and watching for patterns or changes is valuable information wherever you are in your life, and these tests give you a baseline or alert you to problems happening right now.

A full thyroid panel may be in order, too. Most doctors don't order this, and in today's world that means missing out on information that could make your path to health much shorter. If you are 50 years or older, thyroid dysfunction is common, so you should demand a full panel, particularly if you are experiencing chronic symptoms like constipation and/or bloating. Constipation is a classic symptom of hypothyroidism, yet most doctors who evaluate thyroid function do so by only checking thyroid stimulating hormone (TSH) levels. TSH is the hormone that tells the thyroid gland to produce more or less thyroid hormone.

> **Hormonious Point:** TSH levels fluctuate throughout the day, but more importantly, this single marker doesn't reflect how much thyroid hormone is being produced and utilized in the body or whether an excess of antibodies has developed because TSH is produced by the pituitary gland, not the thyroid. The pituitary is the master gland getting direction from the brain, and then directing other glands to produce hormones.

If the lab work from your annual visit is not yielding answers to your chronic symptoms, functional lab testing is a terrific tool to consider in your quest to understand what is going on, even before a condition is diagnosed. Why are your symptoms happening? While conventional lab testing may shed some light on any developing patterns, functional lab testing offers an opportunity to go deeper and assess various systems like the hormone, immune, digestion, detoxification, energy production, and nervous systems. As an example, a common functional lab test measures hormone levels such as estrogen. What makes it unique, however, is that this test can provide insight into not only the hormone levels but how the body is using hormones. In the case of estrogen, you can learn whether estrogen is being metabolized in a protective or harmful way. Though not always covered by insurance, these sophisticated tests can provide highly detailed information and insight that can get you on your road to healing faster. It takes the concept of preventative medicine to a whole new level of understanding and possibility.

### Functional Lab Testing

If you would like to take advantage of lab testing available from an FM practitioner, you can visit the site www.ifm.org to get started. FM practitioners may be available in your area, but many work virtually. I will provide the names of several FM practitioners in the Resources section. You can also work with a Functional Diagnostic Nutrition Practitioner by emailing support@afdnp.com for a referral.

## Medications and Supplements

These days, most people seem to be taking some kind of medication, whether prescription or over-the-counter (OTC). Most doctors want to know what you are taking, so it's a good idea to have your list ready. List all medications and all supplements, too (even multivitamins). Include dosage, date started, and why you are taking it, to the best of your knowledge.

# Analysis

Once you have laid out all the information, review what you have compiled and ask yourself some questions:

- Do you see any patterns?

- How often have you taken antibiotics?

- What in your family's history resonates in your own life?

- Do you notice any connection between a major life event and coincidental health issues (like headaches, digestive problems, or UTIs) that you experienced? Do they line up chronologically?

- Do you notice any mediators or triggering events that you could do something about now? For example, over-exercising causes inflammation. If you are either highly stressed or exhausted, consider reducing the amount of exercise you are doing, as a first step. Or, if you notice that every time you eat a particular food you get bloated, experiment by removing that food for several days and see what happens. If you have experienced trauma in your life, this is an opportunity to recognize what a contributing factor this may be to your health imbalance.

At this point, you may be having an *aha* moment...or a bunch of them! A map of your own health may already be forming in your head. Your direction may become more apparent to you. This is the beginning of increased clarity and self-awareness about your own health journey.

And just in case you think you are too busy to spend much time on this (maybe you read through it and are tempted to skip right to the recommendations), please reconsider. I get it. Life is full and we all have obligations that require our attention, but without health, the rest of it becomes meaningless.

**Hormonious Inspiration:** Remember the quote at the beginning of this chapter? "Be ruthless for your own well-being." It was written by a 27-year-old woman who died of Ewing sarcoma, a form of bone cancer, in January 2018. Her mission was to inspire her family and friends to take life more seriously. Photos on Facebook reflect a beautiful woman in her prime, carefree and engaged in life. She had the heartbreaking wish not to die because she loved living. Sometimes, facing our demons means appreciating life for all that it is—the good and the bad, the beautiful and the ugly.

What I want for you, and for everyone who reads this book, is to understand that good health is not a destination. It is a journey and one that only you can create. What if you only had a short time left? Remember my prompt above for you to look ahead and see your future self? None of us knows for sure what may happen tomorrow. In that spirit, I ask you to put your cell phone away, turn off the news, and spend a few minutes learning about how your past has contributed to your health, or lack thereof, in this precious present moment. This is the beginning of reclaiming the health you deserve and enjoying it for the rest of your life.

I've been in dark places and I've been discouraged. I've hit dead ends and screamed in frustration from the pain, the anxiety, the sleepless nights. There were times that I wanted to give up. While my mom was in hiding during the Holocaust, she was able to read one book that she had with her, *The Count of Monte Cristo*. She read this thanks to a ray of sun that beamed into the haystacks where she hid. My mom gave me the name, Karen, because it means "ray of sun" in Hebrew. For her, that name and those rays of sunlight were symbols of hope, solace, and a better future. To me, this ray is akin to a flame—one that we each carry inside ourselves. It is always burning, inciting each of us to keep going.

It is this flame, inside you right now, that will help guide you, direct you, and support you forward. Feel that inner flame and let it inspire you to find and capture the life you want. You are stronger than you think, and I am here to help empower you with knowledge to keep going, and to never accept anything less than your birthright: optimal health.

## CHAPTER 2

# GUT MATTERS

*"All disease begins in the gut."*
—Hippocrates

As a starting point in the process of getting to the underlying causes of your health challenges, it's critical to explore the
gut. Plenty of my clients come to me with gastrointestinal issues
or complaining of other vague symptoms, such as stress, lack of
energy, headaches, or sleeplessness, not realizing that a breakdown
in their digestive system was the primary culprit. One of the tenets
of functional medicine is to look at the gut first, so it rarely sur-
prises me that renovating a client's eating habits typically reduces
or eliminates many or most of the symptoms they complain about.
Even seemingly unrelated symptoms may have their origin in gut
dysfunction. Understanding how the complexity of your digestive
system interacts with and serves you and the rest of your body can
shed light on your chronic symptoms and how you may be unintentionally contributing to the dysfunction you're experiencing.

Fortunately, these are the kinds of changes that don't require a doctor or a lab test. They are within your control.

Few of my clients have had the extensive history of GI distress that I have, so if you will indulge me, I will use myself as an example of how disruptive gut dysfunction can be, and how I was able to switch course and take steps towards healing.

When I was young, I was an adventurous eater—junk food as a teenager, exotic ethnic food in my 30s. Talk to any of my friends and they'll confirm my inclination for unusual food and flavor combinations. In time, cheese began to bother me, but for the most part I could stomach just about anything. Then, a few years into my training, I began to experience uncomfortable digestive symptoms.

My brother, who has Crohn's disease, has suffered and endured a lot. By comparison, I thought my symptoms were pretty minor, so I tried to ignore them. The irony did not escape me, though: Here I was, studying health and nutrition, while experiencing some of the very same things that I was learning how to treat: bloating, gas, constipation. Did I have leaky gut? Did I have candida? Or small intestinal bacterial overgrowth (SIBO)? Or something worse, like a parasite? And why was I having digestive troubles at all?

I decided I had an opportunity to be the guinea pig and try healing myself. I began to experiment, first with diets, and then with some basic lab testing. I tried a raw food diet (I felt amazing but couldn't sustain eating that way). I played around with FOD-MAPs,[8] GAPs,[9] and a few other trendy diets (ketogenic, paleo, autoimmune protocols). I then experimented with an elimination diet, and to my surprise, that, along with my own Reboot Cleanse[10] (which is essentially an elimination diet), gave me the most relief I'd experienced thus far.

The process for an elimination diet is removing the most common inflammatory foods for a period of time, and then slowly reintroducing them to determine which ones you may be sensitive to. It can be basic, such as removing gluten, dairy, and refined sugar, or it can be more extensive. For example, you might remove peanuts, corn, eggs, soy, and shellfish. In some cases, the removal may be temporary depending on the complexity and nature of your symptoms and last from a period of weeks to up to six months. For others, removal may be permanent. For me, the primary culprits that sifted out in the elimination diet were sugar, corn, and legumes—I have to be careful with these. That information was interesting and useful and eliminating these foods did help me, but it was not the end of my digestive distress.

In February 2016, my husband and I traveled to Thailand. We had an incredible time exploring that fascinating country, eating delicious foods, and even riding and swimming with elephants.[11] It was an opportunity to step back into my exotic eating habits and away from the self-imposed restrictions that had been so successful but that I wanted to wean myself from. In retrospect, it would be unfair to point the finger at the food in Thailand. Of course, that may have been a contributing factor, but so was swimming with elephants (which turned out to be a bad idea, as you'll soon find out) and returning to eating fairly freely upon our return home.

Several months later, I began to experience intense stomach pain, bloating, and other IBS symptoms. Something didn't feel right, so I decided it was time to do some testing beyond the conventional blood tests (aka CBC, complete blood count) through my doctor's office, and the testing for food sensitivities I had done earlier. This time, I opted for a pathogen test, which analyzes stool for parasites and other nasty guests. I learned I had a parasite called *Blastocystis hominis*, which I likely received from swimming with elephants in their enclosed pool (in which I dunked!), as well as *Helicobacter pylori* (*H. pylori*)[12]. The latter is a common bacterium that feeds on stomach acid (also known as hydrochloric acid or HCl) and can cause stomach ulcers, stomach cancers, and uncomfortable symptoms.

Since I hadn't yet studied how to address parasites or H. pylori in my program, I made an appointment with an FM gastroenterologist. I followed his protocol and began to feel better. The parasite situation resolved, but I still had excessive *H. pylori* and further testing showed that I had a nasty case of SIBO (small intestinal bacterial overgrowth; see page 66 for more on SIBO).

Each issue had separate protocols. With the *H. pylori*, it was a matter of taking various anti-microbials and watching what I ate. SIBO was a little bit more complicated and required experimenting with different diets, as there is no one way to deal with SIBO. In the end, the therapy that was the most effective was a protocol in which I drank a mixture called an elemental diet for two weeks and ate no food. This gave my gastrointestinal tract a chance to rest from digestion and allowed the overgrowth of bacteria to die off. I had energy and felt vibrant. I woke up with a bounce and could feel my body returning to its normal self. The elemental diet worked. Watching over my diet and taking supportive supplements to heal my gut followed. (This will not necessarily be right for you—my situation was extreme—and an elemental diet must be followed under the guidance of an experienced medical practitioner, so I will not discuss how to do that in this book.)

Upon healing my gut, the process of recovering my own health was about investigating why I became prone to these gastrointestinal issues in the first place. I was generally healthy. I exercised and ate well. Knowing that my mom's disease would be challenging for me, I took up meditation. It helped but it wasn't a cure-all. I also had a physician dad who in those days prescribed me antibiotics for the numerous UTIs I got during the stress of law school. Did toxic exposure play a role? Even though I wore a mask, I still fainted after spray painting our basement.

As you can see, there are a number of factors that can contribute to a slow erosion of optimal health, and which by themselves are simply facts of life that you endure but on greater examination provide insight into how your resilience could be challenged. As you read this book, I'll be asking you to develop an extra sense— one that requires you to consider your circumstances, state of relationships, your environment, history, and so on, and which you can add to your FTP. Narrowing in on a root cause or causes of your health issues is a process that requires reflection, consideration, and a commitment to being honest with yourself about your life. All of the information I gathered in my own health history provided a framework and starting point from which to create a direction, and ultimately a protocol for healing.

> **Hormonious Tip:** As you work to restore your health, you will be well-served by finding your tribe of support. Friends, family, and health practitioners can each have an integral role in reclaiming your best you. The process of talking about your health struggles can be a freeing experience and one that can help guide your next steps as you become clear about them.

## Your GI Symptoms

The first step in healing is noticing. Think about how you are feeling in your own gut. While we all get the occasional stomach virus or other GI distress, consider the symptoms you experience chronically, either those that you have had throughout life or those that have cropped up frequently in the last few months. Do they include any of the following? Notice that some listed below do not seem directly related to the GI tract but may be indirectly related. Ultimately, your symptoms may be so far removed that it may be difficult for you to make the connection between your gut and your health. Keep reading to see how important the health of your gut is to your overall health.

## GI Symptoms:

- Abdominal pain or discomfort in your abdomen, especially after eating particular foods
- Acne
- Allergies

- Anger or irritability
- Asthma
- Autism
- Autoimmune disorder, any type
- Bloating, need to unbutton pants after eating, look pregnant after eating
- Brain fog, poor memory
- Burping, frequent or chronic
- Coated tongue
- Constipation, hard stools, difficulty or straining when eliminating, less than one bowel movement per day
- Cramping
- Depression and/or anxiety
- Diarrhea, or more than three bowel movements per day
- Fatigue after eating
- Feeling better when not eating
- Gas
- Headaches (frequent or chronic)
- Heartburn/acid reflux/GERD
- Heart rate increase after eating
- Hemorrhoids
- Indigestion after eating (frequent or chronic)
- Inflammation, any kind (external or systemic)
- Migraines
- Mood swings
- Poop that regularly smells bad

- Sensory issues (being easily overwhelmed, overstimulated, having exaggerated sense impressions, hypersensitivity, etc.)

- Sleep that is not restful, insomnia, frequent waking

- Undigested food in stool

This list is not exhaustive.

Did you find yourself nodding your head that "*Yes, I have that symptom and that one, and hey, that one, too!*"? If you discover things you haven't added to your FTP, go back and add them now. (Remember, that document can always be in flux.) If you have other symptoms not listed above, don't worry. The truth is that it would be impossible to list every single symptom that is associated with the health of the gut. This is just a starting point.

But, maybe now, you are wondering why. Why is your gut so influential to your health? How does it work, and where has yours gone wrong? Let's begin by considering two primary gut priorities:

1. The integrity of your digestive tract is paramount. It should be in good condition with no weaknesses or leaky spots.

2. The vitality of your microbiome is just as crucial. It should contain many diverse species with the beneficial ones outnumbering the pathogenic ones; i.e., the good guys should outnumber the bad guys.

These are key elements, not just for your digestive health but for your big wellness picture because remember—health begins in the gut!

So how do we get there? Feeling the symptoms is one thing but knowing the mechanisms behind them can help you understand what is going on so that you'll be more motivated and knowledgeable about how to correct them. Let's begin by looking at how you are built.

# What's Really Going On Inside Your Gut?

From mouth to anus, envision a long, snaking tube, weaving its way around your internal organs. Food enters at one end, is processed in multiple ways, and its unusable waste products are then eliminated.[13] Your digestive tract is divided up into various parts, including the mouth, the esophagus, the stomach, the small intestine, and the large intestine, or colon. Your small intestine[14] is approximately 20 feet in length and is the primary location of carbohydrate digestion and nutrient absorption. The large intestine, or colon, is where the remainder of nutrients are extracted from your food, and where fiber becomes an important part of the elimination process. This is also where most of your microbiome lives (and feeds on that fiber). Connected to the end of the colon is the rectum. And then, of course, we eliminate from the "tail end."

What happens to the food you eat as it passes through that tube is complex and interesting, but in a word, what happens is digestion. Digestion is the chemical breakdown of food by enzymes into particles (i.e., molecules[15]) that the body can then absorb in order to use the nutrients from food. Actually, before you even take that first bite, your digestive system has already kicked into gear. The sight, sound, smell, and even the thought of food triggers your brain to transmit signals down the vagus nerve to begin saliva production, increase gastric secretions (including the hormone gastrin), and rev up pancreatic secretions, all in the service of digestion. The body is readying itself for the food that is literally coming down the pipe. Thanks to the enzymes in your saliva, food (mostly carbs and a little fat) begin their breakdown in your mouth. Gastrin stimulates gastric and intestinal motility, which are the spontaneous movements and contractions that push the food through the body. This process also stimulates the production of stomach acid (HCl).

**Hormonious Tip:** When preparing food or prior to eating your meal, slow down (aka slowwww wayyyy downnnn) and think about the food to activate the physiological powers of the digestive system and the gut-brain connection. This is the parasympathetic nervous system you are engaging, the part responsible for "rest-and-digest." If you'd like to add a spiritual element, close your eyes and imagine how this food will provide your cells the fuel they need to power you through your day. Some like to bless their food and/or honor the spiritual aspect of eating a meal. Whatever mode you choose, this slowing down is a powerful tool that will help trigger the release of enzymes, gastrin, and pancreatic juices and allow for the process to run more smoothly. If you're rushed and stressed when you eat, these systems slow down the entire digestive process and don't allow for food to transit through in a reasonable time, often resulting in digestive problems, which can then trickle into other issues.

Consider as well the location where you eat. Opt for a stress-free environment that highlights the eating experience instead of one that focuses on things you need to get done or on something mindless like TV. Ditch your car for a park bench. Leave your desk and your work at the office and stroll to a nearby community hub where you can disconnect and enjoy your meal. Some office buildings now provide communal areas for employees to, well...commune in. In good weather, take advantage, and remove yourself from the office environment and get some Vitamin D-stimulating sunshine. The idea is to allow the power and process of digestion to work optimally.

## Stomach Acid

Food next passes through the richly acidic environment of the stomach, so the breakdown process can begin in earnest. Most of the protein in your meals is digested here. Stomach acid is also critical for killing off pathogenic substances like viruses and bacteria, and it is necessary for absorbing many minerals. However, because HCl levels decline as you age, you may become less capable of nutrient absorption and pathogen elimination. According to the Institute for Functional Medicine, half the people over age 60 have hypochlorhydria or low stomach acid, and by age 85, over 80% have it. If your stomach is not properly secreting acid, not only has the chance increased multifold for uninvited intruders (hello, food poisoning, and in my case, *Blastocystis hominis*), but particles of food are not being broken down sufficiently. This can hinder your body's ability to absorb and utilize those nutrients. Note that if you're deficient in iron or Vitamin B12, this may be a sign that your stomach acid levels are not high enough—Vitamin C, calcium, copper, magnesium, and zinc also require an acidic environment to be fully absorbed and utilized.

For example, you may be eating nutrient-rich foods or taking a quality B vitamin, but not receiving their benefits because they're not being properly broken down. If you are taking an acid-blocking medication such as a proton pump inhibitor, it is raising your stomach acid levels (i.e., lowering the amount of acid in your stomach) above the optimal pH range of 1.5 to 2.5. (Consult your physician to discuss your options; acid-blocking medications should never be stopped cold turkey.) To check your stomach acid levels, I provide at-home test instructions in the Fix Its for this chapter. This is important to know because low stomach acid can lead to some serious health conditions, including...

**Any of these could be symptoms of low stomach acid:**
- Anemia
- Bacterial & fungal overgrowth
- Bad breath
- Belching
- Bloating in mid to lower abdomen
- Diarrhea (either chronic or right after meal)
- Distention of the abdomen
- Excessive feeling of fullness or increased incidence of fullness
- Fatigue

- Food sensitivities
- Gas
- Headaches
- Heartburn
- Increased incidence of parasitic infection
- Indigestion
- Malabsorption problems
- Nausea
- Nutritional deficiencies
- Rectal itching
- Sleepiness after meals
- Stomach pain and distress
- Stomach upset after taking vitamins
- Strong desire to skip breakfast or other meals
- Sweat with a strong odor
- Unexplained vomiting
- Weakened hair, nails, skin
- Yeast infection
- And more

After food leaves the stomach and enters the small intestines, it needs to be broken down into smaller particles to be passed into the bloodstream. The pancreas secretes digestive enzymes along with bile from your gallbladder to further break down carbs and fats. Digested molecules can then pass through the gut lining into the bloodstream, then up to the liver for further cleansing and utilization.

**Hormonious Tip:** The best way to build a habit is to do introduce it into your life slowly. Eating mindfully once will encourage you to try it again another time. It may not happen every day or at every meal, but doing it once is enough to trigger your brain to say, "Hey, hold on, this is different than what you typically do when you wolf down your food." In time, your brain will remind you because you did it a favor by reducing stress. Your brain likes it when you eat slowly. The more mindful you become, the more quickly you will feel that inhaling your food doesn't feel good. This will help you do it more. Each time you practice eating more slowly and mindfully, you are building that habit into your brain. And while you're at it, share the love and good vibes by asking your meal mates to slow down along with you—you don't need to order anybody to eat more slowly, but you can suggest that you all make your meal as leisurely and relaxed as possible. As you all pause in this present moment, you can each recognize how fleeting and meaningful this moment is.

## Your Gut Lining and Elimination

Your gut lining, also referred to as the mucosal or intestinal lining, is what stands between your inner world (where food molecules are absorbed and delivered to your cells) and the world of your inner body. The gut lining is comprised of intestinal villi or tiny finger-like projections that line the entire small intestine and absorb nutrients from food. The large surface area of the villi enables this absorption to occur efficiently. Tiny microvilli cover the villi and further increase the available surface area for digestion. Together, these comprise what's known as the brush border, which helps the breakdown of food. In order for digestion and absorption to take place, these villi need to keep waving and stay healthy and intact. After the digested molecules cross through the gut lining into the bloodstream to be assimilated, your blood sweeps the nutrients and particles to the liver for cleansing and filtering, and then they will either be stored or delivered to cells for fuel.

Food that hasn't been digested yet travels down to the colon where the remaining nutrients are extracted or digested by your gut flora (aka microbiota or microbiome—see the next section). Water and important minerals such as magnesium, zinc, iron, calcium, and copper are absorbed into the walls of the large intestines. This is also where fiber plays an essential role in supporting the removal of any toxins and moving the stool out of the body in a timely manner. (If you are chronically constipated, lack of fiber could be an issue.)

If your colon is running inefficiently or not functioning, you can "become toxic" (too much waste hanging around) and malnourished (not enough nutrient absorption). Even if you are eating well and following the recommendations in the Fix Its, remember that your gut lining is also instrumental in determining whether or not you are absorbing the nutrients you need. If you aren't, this may be one of the root causes of your health conundrum, whatever it may be.

## Elimination

It is ideal if you're eliminating (by which I mean pooping) at least once per day. Some practitioners like to see elimination happening up to three times a day. Less than once, however, should prompt you to question and investigate. Pooping, or elimination, is equally as important as the digestion and assimilation of food, and the timeliness of elimination matters. When a slowdown occurs, undigested food can rot and putrefy in the intestines, becoming food for pathogenic bacteria and yeast. Fats can turn rancid and oxidize, and worst of all, toxins that don't get eliminated get re-absorbed and released back into the bloodstream. Not good.

## Transit Time

Transit time is the time it takes for food to be ingested, assimilated, and excreted. It depends on the composition of the meal and several other factors, including stress level, gender, medications, and the health and status of the endocrine (hormone) and nervous systems. Carbs digest the fastest (fruits in particular), and proteins are second fastest. Fats take the longest time to digest. Most people cannot process more than 10 grams of fat per hour.

**Hormonious Tip:** Though many are uncomfortable discussing the topic of stool, it's an incredibly important piece of your health puzzle. Take a look at your poop over the course of several days or a week, and you can get valuable insight as to how well your digestive system is operating. Do you see pieces of whole food? Is it pebbly and hard? A color other than brown? Maybe you drank a beet juice so the color is off, but otherwise, brown(ish) is the standard. Add this info to your FTP to share with your health care practitioner. If necessary, an analysis of your stool via a lab test will provide a lot more information as to the health and function of your GI, such as the vigor of your microbiome and whether there is an excess of harmful bacteria, parasites, or viruses. A stool analysis can also measure opportunistic organisms and antibiotic resistance genes. Immunological markers are used to assess the integrity of your gut lining and whether a gut repair protocol is in order. A simple at-home kit is an easy way to accomplish this. Collect a sample in the privacy of your home and send the boxed vial off to the lab. Depending on the lab, you could have results within a couple weeks.

In the meantime, use the following tips as a stool tool guide to assess the health of your poops.

Ideally, your stools should:

- Have a smooth consistency and be easy to pass.[16]

- Leave no residue. Your bottom should be clean and so should the tissue paper you toss in the toilet.

- Leave no stain or smell on the toilet bowl.

- Span the length of your wrist to your elbow (no, really!), and ideally form the shape of a lazy S.

If your stools are difficult to pass and too seldom or too loose and too often, these are signs that something is going on. Inflammation, dysbiosis (microbiome imbalance), or even food sensitivities are all possible offenders.

# The Microbiome

The microbiome is the collection of good, bad, and commensal (neutral) bacteria that live within and on us, the majority residing in our colon. They are living organisms and include bacteria, fungi (for example, yeast), and viruses, and as a community, they are typically called "flora" or "microbiota." The microbiome is sometimes referred to as the "garden within" or the "gut garden," and if you think about it in that context, you'll want to make sure that you're feeding that garden with gut-friendly foods (as suggested in the Fix Its at the end of this chapter).

Once upon a time, doctors and scientists thought the microbiome was responsible only for regulating our bowel movements, but now we understand how much more complex the microbiome is, and what a vast influence it has on us. Your microbiome affects your entire body, including your brain. In fact, the microbiome is so essential to health that some researchers refer to it as a second brain, and I've even heard some experts ponder whether we are actually being ruled by our microbiomes, as a few studies have demonstrated the effects of certain bacteria on food cravings and even behavior.

The microbiome forms at birth as a baby passes through the birth canal.[17] (Thanks, Mom!) Today, C-section babies are often inoculated with swabs of bacteria from the mother, to make up for what they missed in the birth canal. If breastfed, babies get more new flora, which adds more life to the developing microbiome. Babies who are born via C-section, are not breastfed, and/or whose mothers took antibiotics during the second or third trimester tend to have less vigorous and diverse microbiomes, and are consequently at higher risk of obesity, celiac disease, type 1 diabetes, and asthma. When possible, passing through the birth canal and being breastfed are excellent foundations for infant health.

In adulthood, the microbiome performs many important functions, like generating immunity, competing with pathogens for attachment sites and nutrients, stimulating the growth of the intestinal lining, synthesizing B vitamins and Vitamin K, and even balancing mood and reducing anxiety—all of that on top of its famous benefits to healthy elimination. The microbiome is an essential player in the processes of digestion, absorption, and assimilation.

To learn more about the microbiome, visit the National Institutes of Health Human Microbiome Project site: hmpdacc.org. Their mission is to expand the understanding of the human microbiota, and more specifically, to show how the microbiome impacts human health and disease.

Hormonious Tip: Limit your use of antibiotics by asking your doctor if they are absolutely necessary or if there are alternatives for your situation. If a round is genuinely necessary (such as in the case of a serious or life-threatening infection), make sure to follow the completion of that antibiotic with probiotics to help rebuild the healthy bacteria in your gut, since antibiotics kill both good and bad bacteria. Studies show that probiotic use can be an effective way to combat the damaging side effects of antibiotic use, as probiotics can help restore balance to your gut flora.[18] If your doctor recommends taking probiotics during antibiotic treatment, make sure to take probiotics far apart from the antibiotics, or the antibiotics may render the probiotics useless. (To learn more about probiotics, visit nccih.nih.gov/health/probiotics/introduction.htm)

Hormonious Check-In: Studies are showing evidence that the relationship between the microbiome and hormones are inextricably linked. As the microbiome produces and secretes many hormones—such as serotonin, dopamine, norepinephrine, and even some estrogen and progesterone—some experts are referring to the gut garden as an endocrine gland and considering it as powerful if not more so than the other endocrine glands.[19] In addition to regulating the expression of these hormones, the microbiota can enhance or inhibit the production of certain hormones in the body, thus acting as a sort of hormonal conductor—further proof of the importance of a healthy microbiome.

For example, certain gut bacteria (collectively called the estrobolome[20]) are responsible for metabolizing the hormone estrogen. When particular unfriendly bacteria are present, they secrete an enzyme that can impact estrogen levels up or down, producing either a deficiency or excess in the body, and resulting in an increased risk of estrogen-based diseases, such as osteoporosis[21], cardiovascular disease[22], and obesity[23, 24] Antibiotics, hormonal contraceptives, food and lifestyle choices, food poisoning, and travel to a developing country can all upend your estrobolome, making it dysbiotic. Incorporating a probiotic into your supplement regime and limiting your intake of alcohol, sugar, gluten, and dairy, as well as substances that contain phytoestrogens and/or synthetic xenoestrogens (see Chapter 6), is recommended.

# WHAT CAN GO WRONG?

Unfortunately, many people experience problems with a system that should work smoothly. These problems tend to fall into one of three categories: absorption, barrier integrity, and dysbiosis.

## Absorption

First let's look at absorption. You can eat the best food in the world, but if you aren't absorbing it, that so-called health food won't do you any good.

Poor nutrient absorption causes a cascade of issues, as your organs and cells become deprived of the nutrients they need for optimal performance. The key to successful absorption is the health and integrity of your intestinal lining. Remember that inner tube image? The villi and microvilli along that inner lining can get flattened when the intestine is inflamed or damaged. When this happens, the villi are no longer waving and healthy. With long-term inflammation, they can even get destroyed. This will drastically compromise nutrient uptake because of the decreased surface area for absorption.

A classic example of this problem is celiac disease. In celiac disease, the villi can become completely worn away, because the immune system attacks the small intestine lining when it detects gluten. This is known as villous atrophy or crypt hyperplasia. In addition to a sensitivity to gluten, dairy and soy are other foods that can contribute to this "shag" compression or destruction because the body may mistake dairy or soy molecules for gluten molecules, or may be sensitive to dairy and/or soy in addition to gluten. Figuring out whether there are foods you are sensitive to is part and parcel of the process of determining the root cause of your health imbalance, especially if you are experiencing an autoimmune condition. Maldigestion, malabsorption, and malnutrition are all possible when you continue to eat foods that are not only damaging to your villi, but that may be making their way unintentionally into your bloodstream.

Various other diseases as well as parasitic infections can also damage the villi; e.g., Crohn's, tuberculosis, immune deficiency, food allergies or intolerances, and bacterial or viral infections. The villi can also be damaged because of allergies, other autoimmune diseases, chronic stress, toxin exposure, medications, recreational drugs, alcohol, and junk food—especially sugar. There is a consensus among experts that sugar, processed foods, any food that causes an allergic reaction, as well as nonsteroidal anti-inflammatory (NSAID)[25] medications, can contribute to a damaged mucosal barrier. Let the inflammation go on for too long and you may develop leaks, or loosening of the tight junctions of the mucosal barrier, and that (as you will see in more detail later) can be the beginning of immune dysregulation, which can result in much more serious health problems down the line. Damaged villi also set the stage for conditions of dysbiosis (microbiome imbalance), such as candidiasis, SIBO, or leaky gut (the section to come explains these and other gut issues).

There are many ways that the lining can break down, but the bottom line is inflammation, which can cause not only compromised nutrient absorption but also:

- Damaged blood vessels that can impact protein and carb transport and assimilation

- Poor fat assimilation and transport

- A reduction in the cells of the intestinal lining, also known as enterocytes, resulting in weakened immunity

**Hormonious Aha!** If you have constant cravings for a particular type of food (salty, sweet, crunchy, creamy, etc.), consider that your body may be aching for a nutrient contained in that food. For example, if you tend to gravitate towards chocolate more than seems rational, you may not be getting enough magnesium, either because you aren't eating enough magnesium-rich foods or because you aren't absorbing it sufficiently. If you crave sweets, check your chromium level. You may be deficient or have a problem with absorption. If you crave creamy foods like ice cream or pudding, you may be lacking in calcium, and a craving for crunchy foods could actually be a sign of anxiety. If you're a chronic ice chewer, you may have an iron deficiency.

Your microbiome is another prospective guilty party when it comes to promoting cravings. Those gut bacteria can actually send messages through the gut-brain axis that can trigger cravings for the foods they want, like sweet or fatty foods. An evaluation of your diet and some basic nutrient lab tests are good places to start to determine the root cause of cravings.

# What's the Deal with Gluten?

Gluten is a protein contained in grains such as wheat, barley, and rye. The glue-y nature of gluten is what gives those foods containing it that chewy, springy, dough-like texture (think fresh-baked bread). For those who have the autoimmune condition called celiac disease, eating gluten triggers an immune response that flattens and ultimately destroys the villi. The only treatment is to avoid all gluten completely for life. While the symptoms classic to celiac disease are diarrhea, abdominal pain, and bloating, other signs and symptoms may or may not be gastrointestinal, including headaches, infertility problems, inability to gain weight, malnutrition and all its related problems, and even neurological symptoms like anxiety and panic attacks. Infants and children may become severely malnourished or suffer from what doctors call "failure to thrive." Or, there may be no symptoms at all. An FM doctor can test you for celiac disease as well as non-celiac gluten sensitivity (NCGS). Gluten is most definitely a problem for those who are sensitive to it, but it is not a problem for everyone. "If you are healthy, your intestinal barrier is intact, you do not have a genetic predisposition, and you have a normally functioning immune system, gluten will likely not trigger disease," says Dr. Alessio Fasano, generally considered *the* expert on gluten-related disorders.

However, also according to Dr. Fasano, no one can fully digest gluten, as no human has the enzymes necessary to break it down. While our gut lining generally heals itself over a period of three to six days, for people with celiac disease or gluten sensitivity (and possibly for everyone), the damage does not clear up by itself within 36 hours, especially if you keep eating gluten every day. If someone who has a sensitivity continues to keep eating gluten throughout their life, this is likely a problem and could be an underlying cause of your symptoms.

The key in determining its impact on you depends on how well your intestinal walls close after you ingest it and how your immune system reacts to it. Lab testing is the only way to determine for sure whether you have a genetic predisposition and are sensitive to gluten. If you are seeing a functional medicine doctor, you could ask them about the Cyrex Array 3 lab test or the Wheat Zoomer test. The Wheat Zoomer test in particular is an exciting new development that has a 97-99% sensitivity and a 98-100% specificity. In other words, according to Dr. Tom O'Bryan, a world-renowned expert in the field of gluten-related disorders including celiac disease and non-celiac gluten sensitivity, the test is "right almost every time." Traditionally, people had to be consuming gluten in order for tests to come back with accurate results. This is not so with Wheat Zoomer, which can detect non-celiac gluten sensitivity even in people who are not currently eating gluten. Dr. O'Bryan told me, "I personally do not agree with the gluten challenge 'shotgun' approach. These people who are gluten free should be tested now, to see if what they are doing is working, or if they are getting gluten in some other form. Is there gluten in their lipstick? In their thyroid medication? Their vitamins? Their spices?" Gluten hides in many places, not just the bread-y places where you'd expect.

If you do get tested and you do have antibodies to gluten indicating gluten intolerance or sensitivity, the recommendation is to stop consuming gluten, and to do additional testing to suss out any foods that are cross-reactive to gluten. Cross-reactive foods are those with proteins the body may mistake for gluten and mount the same attack. (The test for cross-reactive foods to gluten is the Cyrex Array 4.) If a gluten sensitivity is confirmed, it may be helpful to test for Celiac disease to rule it out as well.

Alternatively, you could try testing yourself through a gluten-elimination challenge. Skip eating any gluten-containing food for a few days and see if you notice any alleviation of any of your annoying symptoms. However, removing gluten for a meal or a day will not give you complete information. If you really want to know for sure, remove it completely for a minimum of 30 days and, ideally, for several months. You may experience relief within just a matter of days, even if you don't notice any symptoms directly after eating gluten. Over a longer period, you may feel even better. If you remove it and you don't feel better, that doesn't mean that gluten is not a problem for you. The complexity of your presentation of symptoms is unique to you and your genetics, and this could be just one piece of the puzzle. If you really want to get into it and eliminate the unknown, work with an FM practitioner to get to the bottom of your body's relationship with gluten.

If testing indicates no sensitivity to gluten, wheat should be ruled out as a possible intolerance for you as well, as wheat is a common irritant causing symptoms similar to gluten intolerance. Wheat has other potentially allergenic properties in addition to its gluten content. Centuries of hybridization have rendered the modern wheat plant more weather- and insect-tolerant but less digestible. Wheat's unfortunate marriage to glyphosate (weed killer) means herbicide exposure to all who eat non-organic varieties. Even if you don't react to any of those aspects, most people eat wheat in its refined form (as flour), in which up to 80% of the chromium is depleted (chromium is essential for healthy insulin production). Also, B vitamins, zinc, and magnesium, needed for carb metabolism, are lost in the refining process, making the starch in wheat less digestible. Wheat also contains the protein lectin, which is an anti-nutrient, meaning it can hinder nutrient absorption. Lectin is also inflammatory and can be responsible for many inflammation-related health issues ranging from leaky gut to immune issues. The Wheat Zoomer lab is an ideal test for detecting both gluten and wheat reactivity. New studies are being conducted to explore whether gluten sensitivity is a result of a microbiome imbalance. [26]

**Hormonious Tip:** Not all gluten-free foods are created equally. Beware of additives, fillers, and excessively refined ingredients, which though absent of gluten, can still disrupt your blood sugar and crowd out other more nutrient-dense foods. Look for as few ingredients as possible, and consider grain-free options as well, such as foods made with cassava, coconut, or almond flour.

## Gluten + Gluten-Free Items

List of gluten-containing grains, flours, and starches:

- Barley
- Bulgar (bulgur)
- Cereal binding
- Chapati flour (atta)
- Couscous
- Durum
- Einkorn
- Emmer
- Farina
- Farrow
- Fu
- Gluten, gluten flour
- Graham flour
- Kamut
- Kinkel
- Malt (malt beverages, extract, flavoring, syrup, vinegar, etc.)
- Matzah meal
- Oats (including oat bran, oat syrup) unless labeled "certified gluten-free"
- Orzo
- Rye
- Seitan ("wheat meat")
- Semolina
- Spelt
- Textured vegetable protein (typically contains gluten)

- Triticale
- Wheat, all varieties (bran, germ, starch)

Gluten-FREE grains, flours, and starches

- Amaranth
- Arrowroot
- Bean flours (garbanzo, fava, romano, etc.)
- Buckwheat, buckwheat groats (kasha)
- Cassava flour
- Chia seeds
- Corn (maize), cornmeal
- Flax, flax meal
- Hominy
- Manioc flour
- Mesquite flour
- Millet
- Montina flour
- Nut flours and meals (almond, coconut, hazelnut, etc.)
- Oats (certified gluten-free)
- Pea flour
- Potato flour, potato starch
- Quinoa
- Rice (all), rice bran
- Sago
- Sorghum flour
- Soy flour
- Tapioca flour
- Teff
- Yucca

**Hormonious Tip:** Although the terms are often used interchangeably, there are distinct differences between a food allergy, food intolerance, and food sensitivity:

**Food allergy:** A true food allergy is an immune reaction to food and will trigger an immediate response after a trigger food is eaten. Symptoms can be mild to severe and can include a rash, swollen or itchy tongue, runny nose, hives, abdominal pain, vomiting, trouble breathing, coughing, wheezing, or a closed airway. Common sources of allergies are peanuts, tree nuts, wheat, soymilk, fish, and shellfish (but there are many more potential food allergens).

**Food Intolerance:** Intolerances are non-immune reactions to food (e.g., lactose, histamines, alcohol, etc.) that occur when a person lacks the digestive enzyme or nutrients needed to break down that food component. Symptoms can appear as flushing, cold or flu-like symptoms, inflammation, and general discomfort. Common trigger foods and ingredients include dairy, chocolate, citrus fruits, acidic foods (like tomatoes), and foods that contain sulfites, histamines, lectins, preservatives and artificial colors, fillers, and flavorings.

**Food sensitivity:** These reactions are not immediate but can impact the immune system. A gluten sensitivity is a perfect example. The symptoms can show up hours or even days later. They are usually caused by an imbalance in the GI tract that is affecting the immune system. One such problem that can cause food sensitivities is intestinal permeability (leaky gut). Symptoms differ from person to person. In addition to symptoms outlined at the outset of this chapter, food sensitivities can cause:

- Dark under-eye circles
- Difficulty sleeping
- Dizziness
- Ear infections
- Excessive sweating
- Food cravings

- Hives, rashes, dry skin

- Irregular heartbeat

- Migraines

- Muscle or joint pain

- Runny nose

- Sinus problems

- Unintentional weight loss or gain

- Wheezing

Common sources of food sensitivities are cow's milk and dairy, eggs, gluten (from wheat, rye, spelt and barley), soy, shellfish, and tree nuts.

# Leaky Gut

Next, let's look at the integrity of your gut lining, which can be directly related to the nutrient absorptions discussed in the previous section. A healthy digestive tract is a tightly woven mesh of tissue that doesn't allow the absorption of bacteria, harmful foods, or undigested food into the bloodstream. It is choosy in what it lets through, only allowing fully digested nutrients to exit. However, when the tight gaps in that mesh of tissue loosen and widen (often due to damage caused by inflammation), the result is a leaky gut, also referred to as intestinal permeability.

The list of leaky gut causes looms large: low HCl and enzymes, infections, toxins, food allergies, food intolerances, impaired blood sugar control, medications, alcohol, and chronic stress are just a few of the reasons a gut might leak, but the bottom line is usually chronic inflammation caused by any of these issues. When those tight junctions loosen, many problems follow, especially the leaking out of toxic byproducts of digestion (meant to stay in the digestive tract for elimination) and undigested food particles that the body can misinterpret as invaders because they are not supposed to be outside the digestive tract. Gluten and casein, both protein peptides, are common causes of inflammation leading to permeability. Zonulin, a protein activated by gluten, is one of the mechanisms by which this happens. It regulates the strength of that digestive tract mesh and in excess, creates those leaks. Zonulin is considered the biological door to inflammation, autoimmune disorders, and cancer,[27] and measuring its presence in the bloodstream is one way to diagnose intestinal permeability.

Signs and symptoms of leaky gut syndrome vary from person to person but can include:

- Anxiety
- Brain fog
- Depression
- Digestive conditions like IBS
- Fatigue
- Food sensitivities
- Headaches
- Joint pain
- Memory loss
- Skin breakouts and hives (indicating the body is trying to release toxins through the skin)
- Thyroid issues
- Weight gain

Ultimately, full-blown autoimmune disease can be the eventual result of intestinal permeability, as the body mounts an over-zealous attack on those "foreign" substances leaking out of the digestive tract. Anyone with an autoimmune condition should be particularly aware of this problem, and will benefit by tending to the health of their digestive tract (start with the suggestions in the Fix Its section at the end of this chapter).

## Dysbiosis

Finally, let's look at what can go wrong in the microbiome. The microbiome contains both beneficial and pathogenic elements. Certain gut bacteria are known to interfere with and contribute to hormone imbalances, autoimmune conditions, joint aches, psychiatric diseases, and weight loss resistance. That's why maintaining a healthy balance is important. Health problems can arise when the number of pathogenic species or "bad guys" grow out of proportion to the "good guys" (this imbalance indicates dysbiosis). This can happen due to unhealthy eating habits (especially too much sugar), as well as stress, surgery, illness, trauma, and certain medications, especially antibiotics. While antibiotics are useful for killing off bad bacteria, they unfortunately kill off many beneficial flora, too. This could be a contributing factor to your symptoms.

Fortunately, because food matters to the microbiome, and what you eat is within your control, you can tip the scales in the direction you want. The standard American diet (SAD) may be reducing the diversity in the average person's microbiome, but it doesn't have to plague yours. Foods that can disrupt the microbiome's natural balance include those that are processed, high in added sugars, or contain artificial sweeteners or trans fats. Choose natural whole foods and fermented foods instead, to help stimulate the growth and strength of good bacteria. I'll talk more later about the best foods to eat for a healthy microbiome.

Also, don't forget that you want your stomach environment to be richly acidic. If your HCl is low, that's another possible reason that dysbiosis may exist. Insufficient stomach acid means that pathogenic undesirables can make their way through your system and into the lower intestine, where they can disrupt the microbiome balance.

## The Five Rs in Functional Medicine

The five Rs in functional medicine refer to the five steps that are an underpinning of FM prescriptions aimed at addressing imbalances in the digestive system. Practitioners are all trained to use this prescriptive advice. If you are interested in following this very specific approach, I recommend that you work with an FM practitioner to supervise the process. This approach can also be considered for addressing symptoms that may appear to be unrelated to the digestive system since, as you now know, the health of the gut is critical to the proper functioning of all systems in the body and may be the root cause or a contributing factor to chronic health issues including autoimmune diseases such as Hashimoto's thyroiditis, rheumatoid arthritis, type 1 diabetes, skin problems such as eczema and acne rosacea, and heart disease (just to name a few).[28]

In case you are curious or want to learn more on your own, the five steps are:

### Step 1 – Remove

Remove any stressors that are negatively impacting the GI environment as much as possible, including:

- **Foods that you're allergic, intolerant, or sensitive to**

An elimination diet is typically used to determine what foods may be harmful to the individual. It is a short-term eating plan that removes certain foods that may be causing a reaction and inflammation, which are then reintroduced, one by one, while monitoring for symptom recurrence. This helps to discern the culprits causing symptoms. As I mentioned above, this kind of diet can be used for digestive issues or for issues appearing to be unrelated to the digestive tract, such as those that are topics of the chapters in this book (stress, lack of sleep or energy issues, mood issues, and weight problems).

- **Pathogenic microflora, such as "bad" bacteria, fungi, parasites**

Clinical approaches for removing these can include botanical antimicrobials, antifungal medications, or antibiotics. An FM doctor would guide you in this step.

- **Environmental stressors such as pollutants**

We can't eliminate them all, but this involves removing as many pollutants and toxic chemicals from your life and body as possible. I discuss some of these in Chapter 6.

- **Stress**

There are many ways to manage stress. I talk more about this in Chapter 3, and an FM doctor would also be able to help you personalize your stress management.

### Step 2 – Replace

Replace the eliminated foods with foods that are not reactive to the individual, and especially with foods that are nutrient-dense. Incorporate fiber-rich foods to support the GI's transit process and function.

### Step 3 – Repopulate

This step involves the repopulation of the microbiome with beneficial bacteria from probiotic-containing (fermented) foods and/or taking supplements that contain beneficial bacteria to restore microbial balance, stabilize intestinal function, and heal and resolve intestinal permeability.

### Step 4 – Repair

This step refers to providing nutritional support for the healing of the villi and regeneration of the gut lining mucosa with nutrient and digestive supplements, along with plenty of whole, fresh, nutrient-dense foods that are low irritants for you.

### Step 5 – Rebalance

This step includes addressing and upgrading lifestyle elements. Poor or insufficient sleep, insufficient or excessive exercise, and/or chronic stress may have played a contributing role in the imbalance. Getting these lifestyle aspects customized to you is essential for optimal health.

I've talked about a lot of things that can go wrong with the gut, but you may already have an actual diagnosis, or suspect you have a particular condition. If you want to know more about your condition, here is my take on some of the most common GI-related disorders:

## IBS (Irritable Bowel Syndrome)

This is a collection of symptoms and if you meet certain criteria, it is a diagnosable condition. Typical symptoms associated with IBS are:

- Abdominal pain and cramping

- Anxiety

- Depression

- Diarrhea or constipation (or both)

- Fat in stools (oily residue left in the bowl)

- Fatigue

- Gas and bloating

- Headaches

- Intolerance to certain foods

- Nausea

- Sleep issues including problems falling asleep and staying asleep

## Candidiasis (often just called "Candida")

This yeast naturally grows in the mouth, GI tract, and vagina. The problem occurs when there's an overgrowth. This often happens in conjunction with antibiotic use, a high-sugar diet, or in cases of mercury toxicity. *Candida* and alcohol both produce high levels of a toxin called acetaldehyde, so brain-related symptoms similar to a hangover are common: fatigue, brain fog, headache, and nausea. Drinking kombucha, a fermented beverage containing yeast, can exacerbate symptoms and is not recommended if you suffer from candida.

Other symptoms of candida overgrowth include:

- Abdominal pain and/or bloating
- Ear itching and pain
- Food sensitivities
- Frequent cravings for sugar, bread, or alcohol
- Lethargy, feeling drained
- Mood disorders (depression, anxiety, irritability)
- Nasal itching
- Skin issues
- Thrush (an overgrowth of yeast in the mouth or throat)
- Urinary tract problems
- Vaginal itching or burning

## SIBO

SIBO is an overgrowth of bacteria that travels from the colon into the small intestine, which is not meant to house these bacteria. The overgrowth affects both the structure and function of the small intestines. If you're suffering from the typical symptoms of irritable bowel syndrome (IBS), there's a pretty good chance that you have SIBO. SIBO has been shown to exist in a majority of IBS patients and is thought to be the underlying cause of IBS.[29] Though well studied and extensively researched at prominent universities such as Cedars-Sinai, SIBO is a condition that is often overlooked or misdiagnosed. The primary issues that can happen because of

SIBO are nutrient malabsorption due to the inappropriate presence of bacteria in the small intestine where nutrients are mostly absorbed, intestinal damage and permeability, and a decrease in fat absorption and other extraintestinal symptoms. Unfortunately, if SIBO is not treated, it can impact the body systemically. Micronutrient deficiencies from Vitamins B12, A, D, E, and K, iron, thiamine, and niacin are common among SIBO sufferers. Critical to this conversation is the fact that SIBO is an overlooked contributor to some common disorders including fibromyalgia, chronic fatigue syndrome, and even hypothyroidism. Shockingly, SIBO may be present in more than half of patients with hypothyroidism![30]

## GERD or Gastroesophageal Reflux

When food passes down your esophagus and into your stomach, there's a door (lower esophageal sphincter or LES) at the end of the esophagus that should remain closed after food passes through it. GERD happens when this door remains open or loose, resulting in stomach acid creeping back up the esophagus. The LES can get weakened in some who consume too much coffee, chocolate, alcohol, and in particular sugar and processed foods. It also loosens with age.

### A Word on Supplements

Supplements can provide the link between what's missing from our food supply and what we need to attain optimal wellness. They also can serve several different functions by acting as a substitute for what your body isn't producing.

For example, if your enzyme production is low, digestive enzymes can stand in until normal function is restored. Vitamins, minerals, and herbs can be supportive or stimulating, like soothing ashwagandha for the adrenal glands, or echinacea for the immune system. HCl supplements can help to replace low stomach acid. Supplements can help to provide targeted therapy with the ultimate objective of healing and restoring normal cell and body system function.

Any supplement that you take should come from a high-quality source and be professional grade and therapeutic. Always check the ingredient list and ensure that there are no fillers or additives that you may be sensitive to. Unfortunately, many supplements include unnecessary and potentially harmful additions like parabens, artificial colors, polyethylene glycol, PVP, and other undesirables. The quality of the supplements you put in your body is just as important as the quality of your food.

# FIX IT

These strategies are for digestive repair, but truly they are also for whole-body repair. Select one and start tomorrow. Once it has become a comfortable habit, add another one. I don't generally suggest starting them all at once because you risk burnout or feeling overwhelmed, and the last thing I want you to do is quit before you've started. However, if you are an all-or-nothing type, then you could take on several, or even all of them, at once. Let's fix it!

# WHAT TO DO

### Chew Your Food Well

Who among us hasn't inhaled a meal because we got to lunch late and are starving, or because we're under pressure to complete a project so we need to eat fast and barely chew, or just because we are stressed about something? This assault on the digestive system cannot be overstated.

The process of chewing your food is as important as the food itself. Chewing is underappreciated, and when done well, it alone can eliminate bloating, gas, and abdominal pain.[31] Mindful chewing creates a pause. The body doesn't figure out it's full until a 20- to 30-minute lag, once some of those nutrients reach the cells, and thorough chewing also helps the body release more enzymes and

HCl. When there are more circulating enzymes, food is more readily broken down and delivered to the cells. This helps the body feel full and sated.

Once food enters the mouth and chewing begins, the enzymes in saliva begin to break the food down, primarily carbs but also to some degree fat. The digestive system is alerted to prepare as well. Finally, chewing also increases the surface area of the food so that the food molecules will be more receptive to enzyme transformation (digestion).

When it comes to chewing, most people just don't do enough of it. Imagine that the most energy-inducing process in the human body is the digestion of food. By aiding and abetting with a more thorough chew, we actually conserve resources our body would otherwise need when breaking food down later. One of my breakthrough experiences was eating macrobiotically after college. The macrobiotic method is to chew no less than 50 times per bite of food. Yes, it's a lot, but it forces you to slow way down, and that should be the takeaway here.

As you begin to incorporate my Hormonious Tips and Fix Its, you'll start to notice that sixth sense, your "awareness gene," developing. That's what we're aiming to do throughout this experience: Grow that awareness, your internal compass. The more aware you become of how you've been doing things and start to consciously replace these habits with healthier ones, you will make fewer slip-ups and oversights. Start with chewing. Awareness can help you realize: *"Oh, I just inhaled that! I've got to slow down next time and not wait until I'm starving to eat."* Or, *"In an effort to support my digestion and my parasympathetic nervous system, I am going to eat consciously."* You don't have to say it in those words. It's the thought that counts, and the thought is: The next time you eat, consciously chew. See if you can chew your food an extra 10 times more than you would have. Doing it once at your next meal is the place to start.

You can make this a spiritual experience by adding in a mindful moment of appreciation for the food you are about to eat, or even a prayer if this idea resonates with you. (This may be part of how the concept of saying grace before a meal got started.) Then, don't just dive in. Eat thoughtfully and allow your body's digestive system to engage completely. The faster you eat and the larger the pieces of food that enter your digestive system are, the harder your system has to work. Well-chewed food will glide easily through the esophagus and into the stomach.

Here is a method you can follow:

1.  Prepare your eating area so that it is neat, clean, and orderly.

2.  Think about the food that you are about to eat and take in several deep breaths.

3.  Take your first bite of food and taste the flavors on your tongue and the texture of the food in your mouth.

4.  Close your eyes for a moment and think about how this food will provide you with energy and feelings of goodness.

5.  Start to chew your food and do so peacefully and mindfully.

6.  For each bite, count to a minimum of 20.

7.  Aim to chew for longer on each successive bite and take note of how you feel at the end of your meal.

8.  Your cells will thank you.

### Test Your Stomach Acid

There are lab tests that can provide a more reliable assessment than an at-home test. However, they are expensive, and unlikely to be covered by insurance. This method is simple and inexpensive and can be performed at home. Try this if you are concerned that your stomach acid is low:

1.  Make sure to perform on an empty stomach. First thing in the morning before breakfast is a good time.

2.  Stir one teaspoon of baking soda into a glass of water. Before you drink the full glass, think about the breakfast you are about to have to engage the cephalic reflex and get your juices going.

3.  After about 15 minutes of drinking the entire glass, acid will react with the bicarbonate of the baking soda and result in a burp.

4.  Little or no burp? It is likely you have low stomach acid. The following section outlines ways to increase this naturally.

## WHAT TO EAT/DRINK

### Drink Water

Water does a lot more than quench your thirst. For one thing, it is essential for proper digestion. Did you know that without enough water, your stomach won't be able to produce enough hydrochloric acid for breaking down your food? Not only can that predispose you to ulcers and acid reflux, but that undigested food will cause a whole ripple effect of trouble along your digestive tract, like bloating, gas, and stomach pain. Drinking more water alone can give your stomach the best chance at doing a good job of breaking down your food and saving you from digestive issues you might have had if you were dehydrated. Your body needs water for many reasons. Here are a few more reasons to make sure that you stay hydrated throughout the day.

Water:

• Aids in the release of energy from food

• Delivers oxygen to the cells

- Dissolves minerals and water-soluble vitamins, and transports them around the body

- Dissolves waste and toxins and reduces the burden on the kidneys and liver

- Facilitates the movement of feces through the colon and its excretion

- Helps regulate body temperature, blood pressure, and pH levels

- Is a key component of digestive juices

- Moistens tissues of the mouth, eyes, and nose

The cells of your body need the proper amount of oxygen, water, nutrients, and the ability to eliminate waste to function properly. If they don't have those things, they will either mutate, die, or rupture. We all have heard the importance of drinking eight glasses of water per day to keep your body hydrated, but there are additional ways to keep your body hydrated, like eating water-rich foods such as greens, fruit, soup, and vegetables. Soups are an excellent way to boost your hydration. And *voila*, there's a recipe in this chapter.

### Drink Filtered Water

Filtered water is best. Avoid water bottled in plastic if you can. Recent studies have found high levels of microplastics in both tap water and plastic bottled water.[32] The World Health Organization is reviewing the risks of plastic in drinking water after learning that tiny pieces of plastic were found in more than 90% of the most popular water brands. Wondering whether your tap water is safe? The quality of your tap water is dependent on the quality of the pipes, whether lead or copper, as well as what other contaminants it may contain. The Environmental Working Group has created a comprehensive database of water quality reports by zip code.[33] There are many ways to ensure that you are drinking the cleanest, safest water. Purification systems that use reverse osmosis remove both chlorine and fluoride. Solid carbon block filtration systems are also effective, but an additional special filter is required to remove fluoride (fluoride is an enzyme inhibitor that contributes to bone loss and other illnesses[34, 35]).

To determine which filter is best for you, please visit the Resources section for the link to a program that will help you do just that.

### Beware Dehydration

The problems with dehydration are many. I've experienced this firsthand on trips to Israel when I thought I was drinking enough but my body told me otherwise, landing me in the emergency room (twice). There are ways that your body becomes dehydrated that you may not even be aware of. For starters, you lose water by breathing, sweating, and digesting food. During an average day, you lose about 2.5 liters of fluid, which for most people is replaced by eating or drinking. However, if you exercise, if you have a particularly active day, or if you sweat or are sick (you have a fever or diarrhea), you are at much greater risk for dehydration. Here are a few scenarios that can lead to dehydration:

- Alcohol intake (drink a glass of water for every glass of alcohol)
- Drinking coffee
- Heavy exercise
- High altitudes
- Hot or humid weather
- Illness/incidence of fever, diarrhea, vomiting
- Infections of the bladder or urinary tract

You may be dehydrated if you are experiencing these symptoms:

- Dark urine (urine color may also be impacted by supplements you're taking)

- Dizziness or brain fog
- Dry mouth or skin
- Fatigue
- Headaches
- Thirst (usually means you've waited too long)

Being dehydrated isn't just a matter of not having enough fluids in your body. It's also a sign that there is acid buildup in your system. When your body is in a state of acidity, that will work against your cells and break them down.

Side effects of being dehydrated are similar to being toxic. Here are problems that could be caused by or worsened by dehydration:

- Allergies
- Alzheimer's disease
- Asthma
- Back pain
- Headaches
- High blood pressure
- Hunger
- Increased stress in your body
- Weight gain

I always tell my clients to drink a glass of water before they eat or when they have a craving because it may be their body aching for hydration. I encourage you to do the same. Thirst sometimes masquerades as hunger and this quick fix will hydrate your body as well. If you are dehydrated, coconut water (no added sweetener) is an excellent way to replete your electrolytes and return your body to a state of balance. If you exercise heavily, make sure to drink extra for the water you're losing when you're sweating.

How much water your body needs per day ultimately depends on many factors including diet (fresh fruits and vegetables increase hydration), climate, and activity levels. Certain health conditions also increase the body's need for water, including fever, UTIs, diabetes, and constipation. A general rule of thumb is to drink about half your body weight in ounces of water per day; e.g., 65 ounces if you're 130 pounds.

### My Favorite Ways to Get More Water into the Body.

- Add a couple tablespoons of organic lemon juice or freshly squeezed lime juice to seltzer water.[36] Delicious, fresh, and flavorful—makes drinking water easy.
- Combine sliced fruit like strawberries, pineapple, blueberries, or raspberries with muddled fresh mint or cilantro leaves. These flavor profiles not only elevate your water, but your vibration, too.
- Same idea as above but frozen in ice cube trays that can then be added to water. As the ice melts and the fruits and leaves thaw, you get the added bonus of a fibrous, flavorful chew.
- Blend water with ice cubes, a couple pineapple chunks, a squirt of lime juice, and mint leaves to make a slushie.

### Add Fiber

Fiber is manna from heaven for the good bacteria in your microbiome, so adding fiber to your diet at every meal and snack is my number one recommendation to you for improving digestion. Fiber is also essential to the removal of toxins and bad bacteria from your body, and bonus: it helps you regulate blood sugar (discussed in more detail in Chapter 5) and remove excess estrogen (see the following section). I cannot overemphasize the importance of fiber. Removing waste and toxins consistently is as important as what comes in the front end. (Remember: Fiber keeps you regular and one bowel movement per day is optimal. Less than that is a sign that something is going on and should be explored.)

Whereas refined carbs raise your blood glucose too quickly (and transit through the digestive process the fastest), fiber slows the rate at which your body absorbs glucose. This not only helps your energy level stay steady, it also means that you stay full longer.

The liver is an important part of the global digestive process in that it is a clearing and storage house for foods and toxins. One of its many roles is clearing excess estrogen from your body. As part of this process, the excess estrogen travels through the intestines to make their way out of the body. What happens if you're constipated and waste isn't moving through? It gets recirculated. Consequently, any hormone imbalance you may be experiencing could be related to a lack of fiber in your diet. Got excess estrogen? Eat more leafy greens, nuts, seeds, fruits, and beans to keep things moving.

### Soluble + Insoluble Fiber

We need both soluble and insoluble fiber, and most food fiber sources contain a mixture of both. Fiber comes from the structural component of plants. You may be more familiar with thinking of fiber as carbohydrates, though carbs that have been refined will contain little fiber and will also be absent of B vitamins, zinc, and magnesium due to the refining process.

Think of soluble fiber as the substance that dissolves in water and becomes gelatinous, facilitating passage of waste through the digestive tract. Psyllium seed, pectin (as in fruit, like apples), ground flax seeds, and chia seeds are good examples. Soluble fiber provides food for "friendly" bacteria in the colon. As a result, these bacteria benefit the body by preventing dysbiosis and synthesizing B vitamins and Vitamin K. Soluble fiber also absorbs toxins and excess cholesterol from the bloodstream—super important! It can help regulate blood sugar levels, too.

Good sources of soluble fiber include:

- Apples
- Asian pears
- Beans
- Chia seeds
- Flax seeds
- Lentils
- Linseed
- Mushrooms
- Oat bran
- Peas
- Pumpkin seeds
- Sunflower seeds

Insoluble fiber does not absorb water. It remains intact and provides bulk to feces, facilitating the passage of solid waste through the large intestine and preventing constipation.

Good sources of insoluble fiber inlcude:

- Asparagus
- Avocado
- Bell peppers
- Berries
- Bran
- Brown rice or other whole grain
- Cabbage
- Celery
- Eggplant
- Leafy greens (spinach, lettuce, kale, etc.)
- Legumes like lentils
- Nuts
- Seeds

There are many ways to add fiber to your diet. Eating greens at breakfast may seem strange at first, but once you make it part of your routine, it will be weirder when you don't include them. Throwing spinach, kale, or any other greens into a blender as part of your breakfast smoothie will also boost your fiber intake. A tablespoon of chia seeds and one to two tablespoons of nuts (such as walnuts or almonds) will not only provide you the fiber you need, but can add crunch to that smoothie, especially if you toss them in at the end and pulse a few times to chop them in.

Soup is a terrific way to get fiber into your diet and is simple when you use ready-made organic stocks. Make it ahead on Sunday so that you'll have it to take to the office or for when you return home. See my modified Anytime Digestive Soup recipe from my Reboot Cleanse[37] in this chapter.

**Hormonious Caution:** Some people are sensitive to the addition of fiber to their diet. If you're not accustomed to eating fiber-rich foods, it is best to start out slowly, adding in a cooked vegetable here and there. Carrots and zucchini are a great place to start as they're easy on the digestive system and filled with water.

If you suffer from inflammation, SIBO, colitis, Crohn's, or chronically experience digestive upset in general, you may be particularly sensitive to fiber. Slow-cooked vegetables are friendlier to the digestive tract than raw. Use an organic chicken or vegetable stock to simmer them to soft. You can also mash, chop, grate, blend, steam, boil, or braise them to help break down the natural fibers, making digestion easier. Make sure that you don't eat the stems or peels from fruits or vegetables high in soluble fibers, including greens like spinach, lettuce, kale, mesclun, arugula, and collards, unless you blend in a smoothie to break the fibers down completely and pour through a strainer to remove any fibers that could aggravate an already-inflamed digestive system. Alternatively, consider juicing these items to access the nutrients. Onions, shallots, leeks, scallions, and garlic can be irritating to the gut, too, because of the fermentable sugars they contain. And finally, don't eat insoluble fiber on an empty stomach. Rather, combine with foods that contain soluble fiber such as carrots, squash, and other root vegetables.

**Hormonious Tip:** Nuts, seeds, legumes, and whole grains contain phytic acid, which binds to minerals in the digestive tract and inhibits the absorption of them, especially calcium, magnesium, zinc, and iron. Also known as phytates, phytic acid is a plant defense mechanism that protects them from insects, but also impacts nutrient availability for us humans. Phytates block phosphorus availability and inhibit enzymes like pepsin from breaking down protein in the stomach and amylase from breaking down starch into sugar. For you, that means incomplete digestion and the many symptoms that come with that, such as gas, bloating, stomach pain, and constipation.

Also, for anyone experiencing bone loss, know that phosphorus works with calcium to build bones. If you are eating large quantities of these foods and experiencing bone loss, these foods may be making the situation worse.

But you can modify this anti-nutrient, digestive-disrupting effect by soaking, sprouting, or fermenting these foods, which helps to activate phytase, the enzyme required to neutralize phytic acid.[38] This makes these foods easier to digest. Some foods can be soaked for as little as six hours or as long as 18 or 24 hours. Soaking nuts, seeds, legumes, or whole grains in water for a minimum of 12 hours will ensure that you have removed at least a portion of the phytates. Make sure to rinse before drying or cooking and discard the water. The size and density of the food will determine soaking time, but 12 hours is a good default.

Another way to reduce phytic acid, other anti-nutrients, and to increase available nutrients is to grow sprouts. Sprouts are seeds, nuts, beans, and grains that have been germinated with water. Sprouting increases the absorption of nutrients from these foods,[39] reduces phytic acid and carcinogens such as aflatoxins (naturally present in almonds, corn, peanuts, and other nuts), and offers a host of additional benefits: It makes food easier to digest, increases fiber content,[40] and increases protein availability, depending on what you sprout.[41] The process for sprouting is lengthier than soaking and requires changes to the water bath over a period of time (several days or longer), and being vigilant that bad bacteria or mold don't form.

While the process of soaking serves the purpose of making the nutrients of the soaked foods easier for the body to digest and absorb, going the extra step to ferment these foods provides the added benefit of creating bacteria or probiotics your body naturally needs. Beyond the probiotic benefits, fermenting foods reduces phytic acid and predigests foods, giving your digestive tract a break. To learn more about how to incorporate these methods into your life, please check out the Resources section in the back of the book for links to online programs.

### Add Probiotic-Rich Foods to Cultivate Your Gut Garden

The terrain of your inner gut garden, or microbiome, needs tending, especially as we age. Studies show that our microbiome changes as we get older and may be a contributing factor to the onset of disease.[42,43] The easiest way to add to your flora is through food, specifically fermented foods that contain active, live cultures. I've already told you how important it is to add fiber to feed those beneficial bacteria, but fermented foods can help replenish the good guys. Fermented foods are probiotic, containing many species of beneficial bacteria. Fermentation has been used by many ancient cultures to preserve food, promote good digestion, and improve health.[44] The process of fermentation converts sugars and starches to organic acids, such as lactic acid. Lactic acid preserves the food by inhibiting putrefying bacteria and promoting a favorably acidic pH in the intestines, therefore elevating healthy intestinal flora and inhibiting the growth of some undesirable bacteria. It can also potentially enhance mineral absorption, especially of iron, zinc, calcium, copper, magnesium, and manganese.

Some probiotic microbes in fermented foods produce cellulase. This is an enzyme that breaks down cellulose, making nutrients more accessible to the body's digestive enzymes. Fermented tomatoes are a great example—lycopene and beta-carotene bioavailability are increased. Fermenting grains, legumes, nuts, and seeds helps to activate phytase. This is the enzyme required to neutralize phytic acid, so fermenting these foods can make them more digestible.

### Some fermented foods:

- Kimchi
- Miso
- Natto
- Pickled vegetables
- Sauerkraut
- Tempeh
- Traditionally fermented pickles and vegetables (not the vinegar kind)

### Dairy options include:

- Acidophilus milk
- Aged cheese
- Buttermilk
- Cottage cheese
- Kefir
- Plain yogurt with active cultures and no added sugar
- Sour cream

**Hormonious Caution:** If you suffer from SIBO, have a yeast allergy or histamine intolerance, you'll need to limit your intake of fermented foods, as they can be problematic for some. In the case of SIBO and yeast allergies, fermented foods can feed the bad bacteria, making the overgrowth in both scenarios worse and increase symptoms of discomfort. Some fermented foods, like cultured vegetables and coconut kefir, contain histamines, which can trigger a histamine allergic reaction (diarrhea, head-ache, runny nose, and so on).

### Add Prebiotics to Feed the Probiotics

Prebiotics are the fiber-rich foods that beneficial bacteria feed and grow on. When probiotics break down prebiotic foods in the colon, a compound called butyric acid is produced. Butyric acid is the preferred form of fuel for the cells that line the colon, and it serves to acidify the environment as well, making it harder for harmful bacteria to survive. As the fuel of choice for the large intestines, butyrate is considered to have anti-cancer properties and may protect against colorectal cancer. Here are a few recommended prebiotics to add to your diet:

- Asparagus
- Bananas
- Dandelion greens
- Eggplant
- Endive
- Garlic
- Green banana flour
- Honey
- Jerusalem artichokes (sunchokes)
- Jicama
- Leeks
- Legumes

- Onions
- Peas
- Radicchio
- Whole grains

## WHAT TO TAKE

### *Support Stomach Acid Production*

Raw, unfiltered apple cider vinegar improves digestion by restoring and activating proper acidity and also by inhibiting the growth of unfriendly bacteria in the digestive tract. Alternatively, add the juice of a lemon to room-temperature water to induce acid production. Start with ½ lemon and if well tolerated, use the juice of a whole lemon. Both of these options can be taken in the morning or before a meal.

> Hormonious Tip: Hydrochloric acid (HCl) is the main component of gastric acid that your stomach produces and is available in supplement form. However, before you add HCl to your diet, you should 1) perform an at-home-test, as described earlier in the Fix It list; and 2) rule out *H. pylori*, particularly if you have been experiencing digestive upset. Since *H. pylori* feeds on HCl, step 2 is critical. Your doctor can detect *H. pylori* with a simple test.

### *Supplement with Probiotics*

Beneficial bacteria are your true best friends and you can add to them by supplementing with a probiotic. Doing so will help strengthen your immune system, reduce chronic inflammation, and help heal leaky gut.[45] There are over 500 species of bacteria making their home in your digestive tract totaling more than 100 trillion (trillion!) "bugs" (microbes) altogether. According to IFM, probiotics must be taken or eaten regularly in order to maintain the colonization in the digestive tract, and they generally recommend ingesting 1 to 25 billion CFU (colony-forming units) daily. There are many brands available—select one that is organic, as the integrity of the cultures will be intact. Also, it's best to select a probiotic with a diverse population and rotate every few months to create variation within your gut garden. Probiotic supplements that contain good GI bacteria include the following: *Bifidobacteria, Lactobacillus, Streptococci,* and *Saccharomyces boulardii* species. Take your probiotic with or after your morning meal, or according to the recommendation of your health care provider.

### Drink Digestion-Supporting Herbs

Certain herbs are particularly conducive to strong digestion. Use them to make an herbal infusion by boiling one quart of water per ounce of herb. Steep the herbs in hot water for 30 to 60 minutes, or even overnight. Length of time and amount of herb will vary based on what you use. You can drink them hot or chilled over ice. Adding in mint, basil, or sage will change the flavor profile. Popular herbs to use include:

- **Stinging Nettle** (Urtica dioica) has many benefits including building energy, strengthening the adrenals, and encouraging the renewal of intestinal villa. (Winning!)

- **Oatstraw** (Avena sativa) reduces cholesterol, increases libido, and strengthens your nerves. It's also known for improving digestion and stabilizing mood.

- **Red clover** (Trifolium pratense) is known for its properties of stimulating the liver and gallbladder. It also helps to ease constipation.

- **Fenugreek** is known to reduce inflammation, improve blood sugar balance, and aid digestion.

### Promote Gut Lining Repair

L-glutamine is an essential amino acid and building block of protein. It also supports the repair of your gut lining which is critical for allowing nutrients to pass through as well as keeping out unwanted guests.[46] Add **L-glutamine** to your smoothies—it's available in both powder and supplement form. It is not recommended for anyone with kidney or liver disease, Reye's syndrome or cancer.[47]

## RECIPE: ANYTIME DIGESTIVE SOUP

This is a flexible soup you can customize to your own preferences: meat or legumes, the vegetables you like that agree with you, etc. Note that cooking times will vary depending on your protein selection.

Serves 4

### Ingredients

1 tablespoon ghee (butter with the milk solids removed)

¼ cup finely chopped scallions, green part only

4 garlic cloves, minced

2 large carrots, chopped

2 stalks of celery, chopped

6 cups of vegetable broth

1 ½ cups brown lentils or 1 pound of animal protein of your choice (chicken, lamb, etc.)

1 bay leaf

1 teaspoon thyme

Small handful of parsley, chopped

Sea salt & black pepper to taste

### Method

Heat the ghee in a large pot over medium heat. Add the onion and sauté until translucent, 3 to 5 minutes. Add the garlic, carrots, and celery and sauté for 2 to 3 minutes. Add the broth, lentils or meat, bay leaf, thyme, salt, and pepper. Cook on medium-low heat until the lentils or meat are tender, approximately 30 to 40 minutes for lentils or pre-browned ground meat, up to 2 hours for uncooked meat. Stir in the chopped parsley and enjoy.

### *Be Creative with Adds and Swaps:*

- Want to do this soup dairy-free? Swap out the ghee for coconut, grapeseed, or olive oil.

- Any vegetable can be added or substituted in or out. You can be as creative as possible, trying a new vegetable you've never had before. Broccoli, mushrooms, Swiss chard, zucchini, leeks—explore the produce section and see what organic varieties are available. For example, you could chop up bok choy and green onion and toss in with water chestnuts.

- In addition to swapping with meat, lentils can also be swapped with any other beans; for example, chickpeas or cannellini. If you don't want to use dried beans and go through the added step of soaking them, you could substitute organic canned beans, like Eden Organic brand. Drain and rinse before adding to the soup.

- Swap in cilantro for parsley and add a squeeze of fresh lime for a burst of flavor.

- Add a can of coconut milk for a delicious, healthy, filling, and satiating fat.

- Beyond salt and pepper, spices are always a good way to boost and change the flavor profile of your dish. Experiment with small pinches of a spice in your soup bowl before adding to the pot. Here are some spice options for you:
  - Garlic, onion, or wasabi powder
  - Dried thyme, basil, and oregano (or *Herbes de Provence*) or other dried green herbs like tarragon or dill
  - Dried spices like coriander, cinnamon, cumin, curry powder, turmeric, ginger, paprika, or

nutmeg
- o Red pepper flakes, chili powder, or cayenne pepper for a touch of spicy heat

# CHAPTER 3

# THE WEIGHT
# OF STRESS

*"It is not stress that kills us. It is our reaction to it."*
—*Dr. Hans Seyle*

When one of my clients came to see me to get help with her struggle to lose weight, I knew right away that weight was not her
primary issue. Linda complained that she'd always had issues with
her weight going up and down, but since she'd turned 50 a few
years earlier, she couldn't seem to lose weight no matter what she
tried. As we got into it, I learned that though her diet needed some
tweaking and there were plenty of opportunities to educate on the
benefits of exercise and lifestyle health, Linda's primary issue had
to do with stress. What she, and many of my clients, don't realize is
that stress alone can drastically inhibit weight loss, not to mention
predisposing its victims to many other health issues.

Linda was in the process of separating from her husband of nearly 20 years, and she had three young children. What she couldn't necessarily see or consciously acknowledge, I could: The pain of a family disassembling (or reorganizing) can go deep. I knew firsthand that when people are dealing with something stressful, they can become myopic, or too close to the situation to understand what is actually happening in their bodies. How do you separate from yourself enough to see what your body needs or even what's happening to it when you are under great stress?

One way is simply time. Some people get to a physical self-awareness faster than others. Therapy can certainly help, as can a lot of quiet introspection. I'm hoping that by reading this book, your internal compass is developing and you are already noticing the way your body reacts to your lifestyle choices. By adding in Fix Its (at the end of this chapter) like breathwork and/or meditation, you can build your resilience muscle—the one that responds to stress by alerting you to manage it rather than repress it. This "muscle" will become stronger as your awareness grows, allowing you to recognize how stressors in your life may be a factor in your health imbalance, and helping you to determine the remedies and answers that work best for you.

Stress comes at us in different forms, from all angles and directions, and at varied times throughout our lives. It can come from family, friends, work, health issues or accidents, and a million other sources. One of the biggest stressors someone can experience is detaching from a long-term partner. It ranks right up there with the death of a loved one, a major illness or personal injury, and a job loss or relocation. Any of these events can create a cascade effect of issues in your body. Weight loss resistance is one of them.

If you are living a life in which you are chronically stressed, your body is compensating—that is, utilizing the resources that would otherwise be available to you when you really need them for an acute stress situation. It's sort of like digging into your retirement account before you really need that money. If you continue at this pace, it is just a matter of time before you may hit a phase of exhaustion and feel utterly depleted of those valuable resources.

Instead, let's conduct an honest evaluation of the stress in your life and where it's coming from. Then we can create a plan to reduce it. These stressors may be external (like job stress) or internal (like a parasite) and could be physical (like an injury), mental (like a strenuous test or difficult task), emotional (like the loss of a loved one), or spiritual (a feeling of meaninglessness, disconnection, or lack of life purpose).

**Hormonious Tip:** What is causing your stress? The answers to the following questions should go in the Mediator and/or Triggers section of the Functional Timeline Plus. Make sure to add them in if you haven't already.

Are any of these stressors relevant to your life?

## *Emotional*

- Death of a loved one
- Divorce or separation
- Exposure to war
- Grief, sadness, anger
- Job loss
- Mood-altering concern over national and/or world affairs including pandemics
- Moving
- Pregnancy
- Raising children (especially without help)
- Relationship stress
- Threat of or experience of terrorism
- Trauma and/or abuse
- Other

## *Mental*

- Challenging college or graduate program Difficulty with test taking or exams
- Difficulty with test taking or exams
- Financial pressures
- Job-related stress or job that requires constant mental attention
- Multiple or overly demanding jobs
- Over-scheduling
- Parenting

## *Spiritual*

- A feeling of disconnectedness, feeling alone
- Crisis of identity, or not knowing who you are in relation to others or life
- Disconnection with your personal belief system
- Hopelessness or despair
- Lack of purpose or meaning in life
- Moral crisis, or realizing you don't know what you believe
- No association with any religious, spiritual, or cultural tradition, and feeling this lack
- Not knowing your personal belief system

## *Physical*

- Accidents, physical trauma
- Airline travel and radiation
- Chronic pain

- Dieting
- Joint disorders
- Major illness
- Nerve compression
- Over-exercise or no exercise
- Over-exertion
- Pregnancy, especially high-risk and/or with complications
- Poor diet
- Sleep difficulties
- Surgeries

I'm sure I haven't thought of everything, and maybe you could add more to these lists, but the point is that if you have chronic stressors like these and you don't address them, they will likely negatively contribute to your current state of health now and in the future. To get ahead of chronic stress, it is essential to get support. Whether that means support through friends, family, or professionals like therapists, spiritual leaders, or support groups, reach out. It doesn't have to be a big gesture. Start small, like calling a friend or non-judgmental ear and asking for support. For physical stressors, get the medical support you need, whether that means working with a physical therapist (PT), massage therapist, or other professional to heal quickly (as is possible) and well. I'll give you more help in dealing with chronic stress throughout this chapter.

## INTERNAL STRESSORS

Another set of stressors that you may be less familiar with: internal stressors. You don't see them and you may not know they exist, yet they are contributing to breakdown. Some of these internal stressors are a result of chemical or environmental stressors. The problem is that chemicals and pesticides get stored in fat cells and removing them can be a difficult process. (See Chapter 6 for more on endocrine disruptors.)

For example, let's say you ate something that was spoiled and contained pathogenic bacteria. Ideally, your stomach acid should provide the initial defense, killing the bacteria. A sound digestive tract only allows in what it should, and the liver takes center stage as the primary detox station. However, in cases where someone is chronically stressed, the body may not be able to defend against the toxins and food poisoning may be the unfortunate result.

After a while, the environmental load in the system adds up. Considerations like low stomach acid, leaky gut, and an overtaxed liver mean that your body needs support to get the system up and running again.

Here are examples of internal stressors:

- Alcohol
- Bacteria
- Blood sugar dysregulation
- Detoxification insufficiency
- Digestive insufficiency
- Drugs
- Endocrine disrupting, industrial, or other chemicals
- Food additives
- Food allergies
- Food sensitivities (antigens)
- Fungi (pathogenic, like candida)

- Heavy metals
- Herbicides
- Inflammation
- Leaky gut
- Lyme disease (from a tick bite)
- Metal (amalgams) in teeth
- Mold (from within the home)
- Parasites (Did you travel outside the country?)
- Pathogens
- Pesticides
- Tobacco residue/nicotine
- Toxicity, any kind
- Viruses

If you have been wondering what is contributing to your symptoms and your doctor is scratching her head, it's time to consider what is going on inside the body. At a minimum, review personal care products you use on your body (makeup, creams, and lotions, etc.) or those for your home (household cleaning, laundry detergent, and lawn care products, etc.). It's also a good idea to review your home's interior for potential stressors like asbestos tiles, mold, clogged air ducts, etc. These are just a few issues you may need to tackle. Consider any travel you've done outside the country as well. An FM practitioner can get you the help you need to evaluate what internal stressors might be at play and how to resolve them.

## SYMPTOMS OF CHRONIC STRESS

"Metabolic chaos"[48] is a term that perfectly encapsulates what is happening to a body undergoing chronic stress. The definition of metabolic chaos is a negative influence (like stress) having a cascading effect within the body so that symptoms may seem only distantly related to the original negative effect but are indeed related.

In the case of stress, here are some of the symptoms you may be experiencing via the effect of metabolic chaos:

- Acne, rosacea, skin rashes

- Allergies, asthma

- Blood sugar imbalance (metabolic syndrome, "pre-diabetes," or actual diabetes)

- Brain fog, concentration problems, forgetfulness

- Depression, anxiety, mood swings, emotional fragility

- Excessive weight gain or weight loss resistance

- Fatigue, lethargy, malaise

- Headaches

- Hypertension

- High cholesterol

- Indigestion, heartburn/reflux, gas, bloating, IBS symptoms

- Inflammation, pain

- Insomnia, wakefulness at night

- Low sex drive

- PMS, irregular cycles

Do you identify with any of the listed symptoms? Did any of these surprise you as stress-related? Here's why stress casts such a wide net of symptoms: cortisol.

Cortisol, released by your adrenal glands, is the primary stress hormone that you want circulating in your body in healthy amounts. Despite its sometimes-bad reputation, cortisol is an important and essential hormone. You want cortisol to increase when you face acute stress in your life because it helps with survival and speeds healing. However, you also want cortisol to decrease when the acute stress is gone and your body is ready for relaxation and sleep. When cortisol stays high, it is the primary culprit behind the symptoms of chronic stress.

Cortisol can cause different kinds of symptoms based on whether it is too high (your body keeps releasing it after the acute stress is gone) or too low (when your adrenal glands are depleted).

Here are the symptoms of when it is chronically too high:

- Anxiety
- Cognitive decline
- Cravings for carbs
- Decreased bone minerals/density
- Depression
- Frequent infections
- High blood pressure
- Hyperglycemia (high blood sugar)
- Insomnia (that "wired but tired" feeling)
- Insulin resistance
- Muscle wasting or decreased muscle mass
- Poor memory
- Poor wound healing
- Thinning skin that bruises easily
- Water retention
- Weight gain

These symptoms can occur when cortisol is chronically too low:

- Allergies
- Anxiety
- Brain fog

- Cravings for salty foods
- Depression
- Dizziness, lightheadedness (especially when rising from a sitting or lying position)
- Fatigue
- Hypoglycemia (low blood sugar)
- Inability to handle stress
- Insomnia
- Low blood pressure
- Low libido
- Low thyroid function
- Muscle weakness
- Pain and inflammation
- PMS symptoms
- Social anxiety

**Hormonious Aha!** CRAVINGS...do you get these? Chronic stress is a possible culprit. In the body's effort to fuel the brain and body during a stressful situation, it needs glucose. To get more glucose, the brain triggers an increase in appetite. At the first sign of stress, practice slowing down and thinking consciously about what your next meal is going to be. This is no time to indulge your sugar cravings, so avoid snacks like cookies, muffins, or granola bars, as they can worsen the situation. Recall my suggestion in Chapter 2 to drink water first when a craving comes on: Drink a glass of water, or maybe two. Wait 15 minutes and check in with how you feel. Are you still hungry? Maybe you were just dehydrated and too stressed out to notice. Even if you weren't, drinking the water can distract your brain and body enough to let the craving pass.

# THE SYMPATHETIC NERVOUS SYSTEM AND THE HPA AXIS: STRESS MANAGEMENT CENTRAL

But how does this whole stress thing work? Wouldn't it be nice if you could just turn off the stress response with a switch? It helps to understand what's really going on with your hormones when you experience stress, because hormones secreted by the organs and glands of your endocrine system are intimately involved in the stress response. To understand the stress response better, let's look at it from this hormonal perspective.

Imagine yourself enjoying a lovely hike through the woods one sunny afternoon, when suddenly you are confronted by a bear. Yikes, a bear! Your brain understands that your very life is at risk, so it launches a process that helps your body respond to the threat quickly and effectively to maximize your chance for survival. This process, sometimes simplified as the "fight or flight response," involves two separate but integrated systems: the sympathetic nervous system and the HPA axis (hypothalamus-pituitary-adrenal). These systems each signal the adrenal glands through nerve impulses and messenger secretions, respectively, to release epinephrine (adrenaline), norepinephrine (noradrenaline), and cortisol into the bloodstream. The hypothalamus continues to signal the pituitary to tell the adrenal glands to keep producing and releasing cortisol until the threat is gone.

This process has many effects on you, including increasing your heart rate, blood flow, blood pressure, blood sugar, and state of alertness. These changes provide your body greater strength and speed to fight the threat or run away. It's an incredible response system built into your body. Even 9-1-1 doesn't respond that quickly. If you've ever had a near-miss accident, you'll understand that adrenaline rush feeling. Your heart pounds, you're intensely alert, and you can feel your body tense up to prepare.

Your brain's ability to send out these signals in response to threats or stressors is so perfectly orchestrated that you don't even realize it's operating, but when it kicks in, all other systems that aren't needed in that moment (digestion, for example) take a back seat.

Let's take another moment to look even more closely at cortisol, because it plays a key role in this process. Here's what cortisol does, in a perfect world:

- Helps to manage acute stress (as described above)
- Is highly anti-inflammatory (which is why it is often used in corticosteroid creams used to treat inflammatory or skin conditions)
- Helps regulate blood sugar
- Aids digestion by stimulating gastric acid secretion
- Regulates blood pressure
- Metabolizes carbs, fat, and protein, increasing blood sugar for energy if it drops too low

The problem arises, as I've mentioned, when we have either too little or too much cortisol in our systems. From an evolutionary perspective, the stress response helped us survive and combat short-term stress, but our bodies haven't adapted to dealing with chronic stress. The HPA axis is tightly regulated by a feedback mechanism, such that the flow is never more than needed and the adrenal gland is signaled to stop secreting when the threat is gone to maintain a balance. But when the HPA axis (and the sympathetic nervous system) are continually activated over the long term, they can get "stuck" in overdrive as the body perceives non-life-threatening conditions (high-pressure workloads, over-packed schedules, constant business, Covid impact) as stress, and this can damage the body and lead to disease. We are not meant to experience stress constantly. And since the stress response system uses the same mechanisms (cells, organs, pathways, and so on) as the body's non-stress system, normal metabolic functions suffer over time because the body is in a constant state of alert and unable to return to its regular functioning.

Here are some of the negative effects of excessive long-term cortisol levels:

- Cortisol is catabolic, meaning that over time, it breaks down parts of the body, like muscle tissue and bone (which can raise your risk of osteoporosis and fractures), in order to support its needs. One of its needs is to raise blood sugar and it does this by accessing the amino acids (protein) in the muscle.

- Cortisol suppresses the immune system and interferes with wound healing.

- Recall that mucosal layer in your digestive tract? Chronic stress can impact the production of sIgA (secretory immunoglobulin), and thus, the integrity of the gut lining, predisposing you to dysbiosis and leaky gut and escalating the risk for gastrointestinal infections and infestation by pathogens.

- Cortisol impairs learning, inhibits memory retrieval, elevates blood pressure, and disrupts sleep by suppressing melatonin, the sleep hormone.

- Have you noticed an increase of fat around your middle section? High levels of cortisol reduce calcium absorption and bone formation, and increase abdominal fat. This visceral fat is known to be a contributor to insulin resistance and diabetes, and is pro-inflammatory, which increases cortisol, too.

Stress is a natural part of life and handling a certain level of stress is to be expected. However, we haven't adapted to dealing with chronic stress with an HPA axis that is continuously engaged. In other words, if your body is in a constant state of feeling it's in a life-threatening situation and the body systems respond accordingly, that means that other systems that you rely on, your digestive system as an example, but your health in general, can be genuinely impacted.

Keep in mind—your system engages when a threat is perceived. It doesn't have to be a bear or even something that you see. It can be something happening in your life that gives rise to a primal fear that sets the wheels in motion. And when it's chronic, the negative feedback loop that curtails the production of stress hormones under normal circumstances can become "unhinged" so that the flow continues. Recognizing what the triggers in your life could be is step one in untangling the system and tackling the stress response (start with the Fix Its in this chapter). Keep in mind that even if everything is going swimmingly in your life, you may be impacted by things that are happening internally, or by things that are happening to others, like your children, parents, friends, or loved ones. In psychology, this is known as systemic stress. If your spouse or life partner is ill, struggling, or in a bad place, there is an impact on you as well. Continue to build up that resilience muscle by finding time each day to disconnect and focus on your breathing (among other strategies mentioned at the end of this chapter).

**Hormonious Tip:** Cortisol secretion follows a diurnal pattern. This means that it is highest in the morning when you wake up, and over the course of the day it slowly drops. It reaches its lowest point at night, so you can go to sleep. This is when melatonin kicks in to aid the sleep process. Cortisol and melatonin oppose one another, so cortisol must decrease in order for melatonin to increase. To support these hormones operating at the times they are designed to, create a morning routine to support cortisol and a nighttime routine to support melatonin.

(See Chapter 4 for more information on melatonin and creating a sleep culture routine.)

One thing to try: When you wake up in the morning, create a stretching practice while you're still in bed, stretching your toes and feet as far as they can go. Do the same with your arms, adjusting your body so that you can lengthen your torso. If it's more comfortable for you, do this right after you get out of bed on a carpeted floor or mat. Incorporating a brisk morning walk outside in fresh air before you're off for the day will also help to get your joints moving, set your mood, and support your circadian rhythm.

**Hormonious Check-In:** Curious what your perceived levels of stress are? You could test it by using the Perceived Stress Scale, developed by psychologist Sheldon Cohen. To do this test, you will indicate how frequently you have experienced certain feelings related to stress in the last month. Scores around 13 are considered average; 20 or higher are considered high stress. The Social Readjustment Scale is another measure. It lists 43 major stressful life events. These stressful events have been correlated with a higher risk of illness. A score of 300 or above = 80% chance of illness within the next two years; 151-299 = 50% chance; and 150 or less = 37% chance. Links to both are in the Resources section.

## Allostasis: The Goal

Remember that scary bear that got your cortisol pumping? Let's say that bear has gone back to the river to catch fish, and you are safe and sound. Once that happens and the threat is eliminated, your body should return to a state of "allostasis." Allostasis means "stability through change," and it is a term used to describe the optimal functioning of the HPA axis because it's a dynamic system that is always adapting in the face of ever-changing conditions and in response to stressors. And sure enough, hormones are involved. One mechanism for assisting in this ever-changing balancing act is DHEA. DHEA (dehydroepiandrosterone) is a steroid hormone made naturally in the body. It acts as a balancing agent to cortisol so that when cortisol is revved up too high, DHEA should increase to act like a refilling station. Whereas cortisol in excess has the effect of breaking muscle down, DHEA helps rebuild you from the catabolic impacts of cortisol. This hormone is responsible for promoting growth and repair of proteins, especially muscle tissue. It is also the precursor to estrogen and testosterone. DHEA and cortisol should be in a nice balance to one another in lab results. Depressed DHEA levels are an early warning sign of adrenal or HPA-axis dysfunction and may lead to numerous chronic stress-related disorders.

Allostasis was my goal for Linda, the client I told you about at the beginning of the chapter. Linda is a textbook example of a Type-A personality. She runs on adrenaline. She also is the primary earner in her family, so she shoulders the financial responsibility. It wasn't until her body began reporting back to her that *it just couldn't take it anymore* that she knew she needed to get help. Her doctor's simple solution to "work less" wasn't sufficient or realistic. She needed more direction. What worked in her favor was her openness to examine how she could incorporate simple shifts in her life that would support and replenish her.

Our plan involved upgrading her foods, honoring her sleep, and examining all the pieces of her life and how they were either depleting or adding to her wellness. She constructed a meditation space in her office with a floor cushion. Coworkers know she's meditating and don't disturb her when she hangs the "Shhh, I'm meditating" sign on her door.

You can do the same kinds of things to get on top of your stress so that *you* are in control instead of the other way around. And, as Dr. Hans Seyle wisely pointed out (in the quote at the beginning of this chapter), your reaction to chronic stress is what is most damaging. Now that we have strategies in place, Linda feels much better and she reports that she is steadily losing that weight that wouldn't budge before. Victory!

If you're a human being, a certain level of stress is unavoidable. Whether working to support yourself and your family, managing a home, caring for children and/or elderly parents, balancing financial obligations and making time for relationships and social activities, or handling an assortment of other stressors, life can be unwieldy. Throw in a job loss, a death in the family, an accident or an injury, and suddenly it can all seem unmanageable. But again, it's how we face stress and handle it that determines whether it will upend our balance and set us on a path of illness or disease.

But let's be realistic. While I'm a strong believer and proponent of positivity, the concept of "just think positive and all will be okay" can be frustrating and can also mask the very real struggles you may be facing. Here's the truth: You will always have stress. It's part of life. But you can sift through your stress. You can lessen it. And most importantly, you can learn to manage it, so when (not if) it happens, you will be ready. One of the best ways to start that I know of is to build a reservoir of calm by learning to meditate. If you commit to a regular practice of meditation (or just stopping, sitting, and breathing deeply, or other similar techniques) like you commit to brushing your teeth daily, you will notice a difference, I promise. If the idea of setting up a daily meditation is beyond your comfort level, then start with my favorite 4-7-8 breathing technique (described later in this chapter). If you are ready to add breath work or meditation into your life, the changes you experience will be life altering.

Hormonious Check-In: Are you stress eating? The connection between your emotions and your eating may be quite direct, especially when you are under pressure and in a high-intensity work situation, high-stress state, or other emotionally depleting circumstance. Binge eating or just chronic overeating of soothing but unhealthy foods can feel temporarily relieving, but there are two important points to consider:

1. The obvious one is the implication on your health goals and reversing the downward trend of any chronic symptoms you are experiencing. Soothing yourself with food may offer momentary relief but can worsen your symptoms, making your road to better longer and harder.

2. Perhaps even more importantly, addressing the "why" of this response will be more useful and powerful, and ultimately inspire you to change your course.

If you often eat to fill an uncomfortable space, void, or emptiness, and eating seems to fix it, know that you are experiencing something akin to a drug response, such as an opiate experience. The science is strong on sugar's opiate-like qualities.[49] Try taking a moment between craving and eating to consider: Are you wanting to eat in a calm state, with joy and satisfaction? Or are you compelled to eat to dull the bad feelings related to a bad situation or to a situation that is outside of your control? Ask yourself the quintessential question: Why am I eating this right now? Don't eat until you can feel good about the answer to this question. This simple practice can help you gain valuable insight into your behavior and how it is intimately tied to your choices. It's all in the service of increased body awareness.

If you are in a high-stress state and tend to go for foods that will leave you depleted, here are a few more ways to get on top of this:

1. Keep healthier options nearby so that you can reach for these instead.

    a. Drink water first. When in a high-stress situation, drinking water provides you with two benefits. One, you need to swallow water, which forces you to take deep breaths in between (so you don't choke), activating the very effective stress management technique of deep breathing. Two, drinking water quenches your body's thirst, hydrating you and preventing the dehydration that can cause stress in the body. This water break will help you put a pause on reaching for a no-friend-to-you food and give you the opportunity to slow down and think about what you are doing.

b. Reach for a fresh fruit or veggie instead of junk food. Always (always, always) have fresh cut vegetables easily available. If you are pinched for time, purchase pre-cut on Sunday and bring them with you to your office with an ice pack (if refrigeration isn't available).

c. A square or two of dark chocolate (80% or higher is ideal), eaten slowly, letting the chocolate melt on your tongue, might satisfy you when you're in that uncomfortable space and want sugar. Dark chocolate contains nutrients such as magnesium, iron, and potassium, unlike many other sweet treats. Alternatively, pair a square with a tablespoon of sunflower seed butter. The rich decadence of the chocolate combined with the salty, satiating sunflower seed butter will refocus your attention to the present and happify your cells.

2. If you do end up eating that yuck thing, forgive yourself and move on. Let it go this time, but if it continues, you may want to consider outside support such as a therapist to help you dig deeper.

## FIX IT

### *What to Do*

Overcoming your stress in a meaningful way begins with identifying your stressors and creating a strategy for handling and facing them. If you haven't yet done so, create a list of stressors that you are dealing with (check your FTP for reminders). Review possible ones listed at the outset of this chapter, and if you discover new ones, make sure to add them in. As you move through this Fix It section, consider that each of these strategies is designed to get you thinking about and building more calm and resilience into your body, brain, and life.

### Take Space for Yourself

Clear your mind and think about what you want your life to look like. If you are stressed beyond capacity, your body will do what it can until it can't. Honor yourself by giving your body this break, during which you are not dealing with anyone else's needs and problems. This means setting aside time every day to reflect upon your day, how you are feeling at this moment, and being present with your thoughts.

The optimal time to do this is before a meal—you'll manage stress better, be less prone to stress-eat, and enjoy the added benefit of slowing down before your meal to let your digestive juices kick in (three benefits with one action = efficient!). Take several minutes to think about how your day is going: What is going well, and what could use your extra attention? You can do this outside of mealtimes, too (the more often, the better). Take time to breathe and reflect. I recommend that you spend at least 10 to 20 minutes in total checking in with your state of mind each day.

Add in additional time on the weekend when you may have more of it. Ask yourself if you are spending time doing the things that fill your soul, that make you smile. Maybe make a dream list of things you want to be doing in your life. Writing? Painting? Acting? Fly fishing? Starting your own business? Becoming an activist? Volunteering to help animals or children or the environment? Pleasurable as well as meaningful activities reduce stress.[50] Even thinking about pleasurable activities reduces stress!

So think away.

### *Curate Your People*

The most common stressors arise out of family and work relationships, but you can take steps to correct these:

- Minimize interactions, when possible, with a family member who is difficult, doesn't understand or support you, or with whom you derive little enjoyment. If it is impossible to do so, take some time out to consider these questions: What is it that you would want to change if you could? Are there ways to start moving in this direction? How can you reduce the amount of time you spend with that family member? Or, alternatively, how can you find effective support to help guide you through the process of improving and strengthening that relationship so it is less stressful?

- Evaluate your work environment. Dealing with a co-worker or boss whose personality is incongruous to yours can make work stressful or even intolerable. Take space from these toxic environments to evaluate whether you can afford to find another job. What would be involved? Who could help with this? Are you interested in another career altogether? What would happen if you change nothing in your circumstances? Are there ways to stay in your job and make the situation better? You may find support in the human resources department of your employer.

- Simply spend less time with any person(s) who is unable to provide the kinship and support that you need at this time, or who negatively influences you and brings your energy down. You may not even know or be able to define what exactly this person does that depletes you, but if you notice that when you spend time with this particular person, you don't have a good feeling, heed your own instinct. This is important information for you to add to your knowledge bank. Especially take a vacation from anyone who is verbally or emotionally abusive or doesn't have your back, if you can. If you can't, make longer-term plans to change your situation. Ask for help if you need to. Time is too short and you are too important to waste.

- Engage support wherever you can. A therapist, friends, a religious or spiritual leader, a community network, or a career guidance agency could each play a role in moving you through and out of stressful environments, or help you find ways to improve them.

- Spend more time with those who love you, support you, and want to see your inner flame glow and grow. These are the people who can help lift you up and support your road to physical and emotional wellness. This is your tribe.

- Work on building your inner resolve and calm so that as you continue to face that trying relationship or situation, your reactions reflect inner peace. The work that you do will also support your body's build-up of resilience.

### Revise Your Self-Talk

You spend a lot of time with yourself. Hopefully, the majority of that time is positive, but for many people, alone time consists of self-berating and misery. The words you use and the messages that you repeat to yourself about yourself can be not only false but damaging to your self-esteem, confidence, and health. I always ask my clients to begin paying more attention to the things they tell themselves in their own heads. What do you say to yourself or think about yourself when you wake up in the morning? When you look in the mirror? When you drive your car or ride the train?

Do you notice any patterns or any negative self-talk? If so, it's time to upgrade your thoughts and do a revamp—a renovation of sorts, to align your thoughts with more positive intentions for your own health and success. Here are some ideas:

- **Start an I Am list.** This is a list of things you strive to be—descriptions of your best self, worded as if they are true (and often you may discover they already are). For example: I am strong. I am joyful. I am healthy. I am confident. I am beautiful. I am intelligent. Be as specific as you like. It doesn't matter for the moment if you're not feeling these things. What matters is that you want to be feeling these things. It's like smiling when you're not happy. Over time, smiling can trick your brain into actually feeling happier.[51] This exercise will help you create more happiness in your life, which can also support your longevity.[52] Some of my clients put their I Am list on a postcard and keep it on the nightstand, in their purses, or on their bathroom mirrors. Do what feels right to you, but read your list every morning, throughout your day, and at night as you're readying yourself for bed. Get it in your head!

- **Create a daily intention.** Every day, tell yourself that you intend to... (fill it in), and try to be as specific as possible so that you can imbue yourself and your day with that message. Express it as often as you can throughout the day. Here are some examples:
  - Today, I intend to focus on the positive.
  - Today, I intend to smile and find humor where I can.
  - Today, I intend to be kind to someone.
  - Today, I intend to be aware of any negative

thoughts that enter my mind.

- o Today, I intend to abstain from being judgmental towards others.
- o Today, I intend to take a deep breath and pause before responding to someone with negative energy.

Do you spend time ruminating about interactions with others or worrying about something outside of your control? Note the operative "outside of your control" element. If there's something you can do to improve a situation, go for it. If not, and it is preoccupying your brain space for an inordinate amount of time, or preventing you from doing anything else, take a piece of paper and write about it. Every thought you have should go onto that sheet. Once complete, rip it up and move on. Find an activity that brings you joy and move into that space. The best way to get over something is to physically move your body into another space and activity. If you find this too difficult, a professional therapist who practices cognitive behavioral psychology can help.

### Face and Deal with Any External Stressors

If you have suffered from an accident, illness, or other physical injury, enlist support for purposeful healing by way of professionals you may not have considered in the past. Here are several healing modalities that can shorten your healing journey and address other stressors as well.

- Acupressure
- Acupuncture
- Ayurvedic Medicine
- Biofeedback
- Chiropractic
- Guided imagery or visualization

- Hypnosis

- Massage therapy

- Naturopathy

- Neurofeedback

- Physical therapy

- Reflexology

**Hormonious Tip:** Neurofeedback is a treatment for modifying brainwaves to bring the brain to optimal working function. This modality is one of the more successful methods for reducing symptoms of anxiety and increasing attention and focus. Given that stress is directly related to anxiety, both as cause and effect, reducing anxiety through neurofeedback can have a direct impact on the way you cope with stress and incorporate it adaptively into your life. Several sessions are needed to train the brain to balance between the different brain waves. This drug-free treatment is non-invasive and pain-free, although it may not be covered by insurance.

### Get Rest

Ensure that your body gets the proper rest it needs to recover from the destructive nature of chronic stress. You'll find sleep tips in Chapter 4. In addition to the activities described next, call on the 4-7-8 breathing technique explained a little later in this chapter for times when you wake up in the middle of the night. For optimal effectiveness, practice it consistently.

### Breathe Well and Meditate

Build calm into your life and incorporate these science-backed restorative activities that will make a difference internally. These not only help to reframe your state of mind but will help to balance your hormone and immune function. The evidence is clear that mindfulness alters brain chemistry, reduces anxiety, and increases positive affect.[53] It also improves depression and pain.[54] Select an activity that resonates with you and do this practice daily. Like exercise, this is a habit that you need to create for yourself. Meditation is a means of relaxing the mind and the body for purposes of creating calm while elevating mood. It's the best bang for your buck to add to the resilience bank. There are many ways to meditate and to achieve a state of mindful presence and calm. Interrupting thoughts at the outset of your practice and onward are normal and expected. Here are a few options for you to start, and which are current at the time of this writing:

- There are many meditation apps that can help you get the process started. Find one that you like to get going.
  - Headspace is free and good for beginners, offering 10-minute meditations.
  - Insight Timer is home to almost four million meditators and offers free guided meditations, music tracks, talks, and courses.
  - The Mindfulness app is free and offers a five-day guided meditation program to get you started, along with guided and silent timed meditations from three to 30 minutes.
  - The Aura app provides a daily three-minute moment for yourself and ties it to an existing habit, like after showering, exercising, or eating breakfast. You can customize it at the time you want to do it, too.
  - The Calm app offers Daily Calm. You can use it for free or pay an annual fee for expanded offerings.
- Jon Kabat-Zinn, the founder of the Stress Reduction Clinic at the University of Massachusetts Medical School, has created a four-part home training course

entitled "Guided Mindfulness Meditation." You can find this on Amazon or at other online retailers.

- Mindfulness meditation is a way for you to tune into your thoughts and feelings and anchor yourself in the present. This process can help you increase self-aware-ness and refine your internal compass.

  o To get into a state of mindfulness, find a comfortable and quiet spot where you can pay attention to your emotions and physical feelings. Are you happy? Sad? Is your body experiencing any tension or stress? Pay attention to those areas and see if you can relax them. Take a deep breath in and then out. Do this while focusing on any area of your body that feels tense. Consider if there is something in particular contributing to these feelings. Keep returning to focusing on your breath. Let thoughts of your day and interactions float by and resume listening to the sounds of your inhale and exhale if you get distracted. When you are ready, bring your awareness back to its regular state and carry on with your day.

- Gratitude journaling is an activity to ground you in recognizing and appreciating things that are good in your life. Robert A. Emmons, Ph.D., a leading scientif-ic expert on gratitude, believes that expressing grati-tude affirms goodness in your life and has emotional and physical benefits. There are several ways to benefit from this activity.

  o Every evening, write three things for which you are grateful. It can be as simple as 1) I have arms to hug with; 2) I have a bed to sleep in; 3) I have breath. You can keep these recorded in a journal and add to it daily, nightly, or whenever you are in a negative mood. Expressing feelings of gratitude in writing may help lighten your mood and change the course of any negative thoughts that may be attached to it.

o   Expressing thanks is incredibly therapeutic. Write a letter to someone who has helped you in your life. Explain in detail how this person has made an impact on you and describe the inspired change or direction you took. You can either share this letter with this person or simply keep it for yourself.

**Hormonious Jewel:** In my training at IIN, I learned an incredibly useful breathing technique from Dr. Andrew Weil. I recommend this to my clients who are particularly stressed, and it is extremely effective when done consistently. Practice this simple breathing system daily and make it a regular part of your life. Once it becomes a habit, you'll be able to use this tool any time you get stressed, whenever you can't fall asleep, or to help you return to sleep if you wake up in the middle of the night.

**Inhale to a count of four. Hold to a count of seven. Exhale to a count of eight.**

Do four cycles of this every morning when you wake up and four cycles when you go to sleep.

You may notice an immediate calming effect when you do it. As in right now. Try it. I'll wait. Keep doing it. 4-7-8 has been life-changing for me and for every client, friend, and person I share it with. The only person I ever knew who said it didn't work for her admitted that she never practiced it regularly. You must do things consistently for them to make a difference. You are building your calming muscle here.

### *Exercise*

The benefits of exercise to reduce stress are well-documented. Low physical activity is a major contributing factor to overall poor health; without exercise, you are adding fuel to the fire.

> **Hormonious Caution:** If you are overly stressed, intensive exercise is not good for you. Recall that cortisol breaks down muscle tissue. High-powered exercise on top of other stress puts your body into a double inflammatory state. If highly stressed, aim for more calming exercises, such as yoga, light stretching, and walking. (But don't use this as an excuse to skip exercise altogether!)

### *Spend Time in Nature*

Nature heals. The more you can expose yourself to it, the better. A simple walk in a park, forest preserve, or even just around your neighborhood, can help you find calm and fill you up emotionally and spiritually. If you're like most people, you probably don't spend a lot of time outside. In a recent survey, most people reported that nearly 87% of their time is spent inside (home, office), with an additional 6% spent in their cars.[55] Make spending time in nature a habit by adding it into your weekly schedule. Use the hashtag #NatureWalk to share how you are healing in nature today!

Other ways to connect with nature are to buy some plants and put them in nice pots to bring nature inside your home or workplace. The process of getting your hands and nails into soil, connecting with literal earth, and creating a soothing arrangement for your space that you made yourself can be incredibly calming and satisfying. One of my favorite summertime activities is potting a plant. A dear friend and expert landscaper taught me the key elements in a successful potting experience: spill, fill, and thrill. Spill plants are those that hang over the side. Fill plants will occupy the center of the pot with their mass, and thrill plants have height or a distinctive bloom. My latest obsession is using specialized plants, such as verbena, pineapple mint, and sage, which I pinch off and add to my water. (If you aren't up to this level of creativity or mess, you could also buy a nice potted plant and bring it home.)

Plants not only help to reduce stress[56] but also purify the indoor air[57, 58] and might even help you be more productive—try putting one on your desk and share with the hashtag #AlwaysBeGrowing to spur others to green up their environment.[59]

### Smell Your Way to Health

I have always had a passion for scents and soaps. They can upgrade your shower experience to a spa one, breathe new life into your car space, or simply support you to shift into a calm state. Essential oils and a diffuser can do wonders for a variety of ailments, but to reduce stress my favorites include: lavender, bergamot, frankincense, geranium, vetiver, and rose. Find one that suits you and carry it with you. A few drops on your wrist can help initiate the process to downshift from a stressful state. All you may need is a whiff from an open bottle. Take in several deep breaths and exhale. Keep doing it until you arrive at your zen place. If you are regularly wearing a mask throughout your day, consider adding a drop of your favorite essential oil to the inner lining to perk up your senses and even your posture.

## REDUCE STRESS-PROMOTING ACTIVITIES

Reduce activities that may be contributing to stress. If you have an addictive personality, playing games online or engaging in any behavior that is raising your cortisol levels higher (for example, gambling, watching the news, or getting worked up over competitive sports) may be counterproductive to your need to curb your cortisol output.

Take breaks from electronics by creating a home base for them along with a self-imposed policy that electronics get put away at a set time every evening. If you have children, you may see the need to set an example, as our children's attachment to technology may have far-reaching and damaging effects we can only imagine right now.

## WHAT TO EAT

### *Eat Healthy = Remove the Bad Guys*

Whether your stressors are external or internal, your road to feeling better must include eating better. Reduce/eliminate the worst offenders, which are the ones exacerbating stress in your body (I will give you in-depth information about how to cut these offenders out of your life in Chapter 6):

- Alcohol
- Artificial sweeteners
- Caffeine
- Gluten
- Refined and processed foods
- Sugar

### *Eat Healthy = Add the Good Guys*

When it comes to stress, healthy fats are your friends. In addition to enhancing hormone and neurotransmitter cell communication, good fats (i.e., natural fats, or fats as they occur in nature, like avocados, nuts, seeds, and olive oil) are a source of energy that help heat your body, drive metabolism, and move muscles. They also provide a feeling of satiety and slow the release of sugar into the blood, thereby keeping cortisol in check.

There are many other great stress-reducing foods, and I'll tell you exactly what food sources to add in and how to do this in Chapter 6, but in short, default to dark leafy greens (spinach, Swiss chard, kale, etc.), beans (black, lentil, chickpea), quinoa, and seeds (pumpkin, sesame, and sunflower) for most of your carbs. They not only provide a serious dose of fiber (your inner terrain will thank you), but they provide you with much needed magnesium, which is a calming and relaxing mineral essential to your nervous system.

As for protein, recall that excessive cortisol breaks muscle tissue down. In addition to balancing out your cortisol with stress-reducing activities, sufficient protein supports muscle development, bone health, tissue repair, blood oxygenation, and basic cell activity. While animal protein (meat, dairy, and eggs) offers the most complete protein (because of the essential amino acid profile your body needs and animal protein contains), plant protein sources can be integrated into your diet as well, such as plant-based protein powders, beans and legumes, and nuts and seeds.

**Hormonious Tip:** Studies have shown that omega-3 fatty acids can help support length and quality of sleep,[60] reduce anxiety and mood disorders, and lower inflammation.[61] Your body needs both omega-3 and omega-6 fatty acids for optimal health. The problem is getting these fats in the proper proportion to one another. While some studies support an ideal ratio of omega-6 to omega-3 of approximately 1:1, others support a ratio of between 2:1 and 4:1. The common ratio in the Standard American Diet is closer to 20:1, so even 4:1 would be a major improvement. Achieve this ratio by replacing your dietary omega-6 fatty acids (from things like meat, too many grains, processed food, and vegetable oils such as canola and corn oil) with omega-3 fatty acids. Here are some ideas:

- Eat dark, oily fish (tuna, salmon, mackerel, and sardines) in place of chicken, pork, or beef

- Choose pasture-fed over grain-fed meats (grain-fed = omega-6)

- Choose walnuts, sesame seeds, flax seeds, and pumpkin seeds over peanuts. Flax seeds have the highest amount of omega-3 fatty acids – 7 grams in ¼ cup compared to 2.3 grams in ¼ cup of walnuts

- Increase consumption of dark green vegetables

• Reduce consumption of processed foods, including fried foods, commercial baked goods, and margarines

# WHAT TO TAKE

### *Herbs That Help Relieve Stress* [62,63]

Herbs that help relieve stress are known as adaptogenic because they create balance within and help regulate your internal communication systems. They don't just stimulate levels of a hormone or suppress levels of a hormone—they actually help your hormone-producing organs and glands talk to your brain better.

• Ashwagandha is one of my favorite herbs to recommend to my clients who are stressed because of its ability to bring cortisol up when low and bring it down when high. It is also effective for anxiety and brain fog and can help calm you down. It works for most people, but not all. Please follow package directions and pay attention to how you feel after you take it. Just because something works for one person does not mean that it will work for you. Many people can tell an immediate difference, but if you don't feel it, try Holy basil, described next, as an alternative. Ashwagandha is available in capsule, tablet, tea, tincture, and powder form. If you are sensitive to nightshade vegetables (especially likely those with autoimmune disorders or joint issues), consider Eleuthero, another great adaptogenic herb.

Safety precautions for Ashwagandha:

- Avoid if you are sensitive to nightshade vegetables
- Avoid if hyperthyroid
- Avoid while pregnant
- High doses can cause GI upset

- Use cautiously with low blood pressure

Holy basil (Ocimun sanctum)[64] also commonly referred to as tulsi tea, is another great stress-management herb. Holy basil is an adaptogen with antioxidant, neuroprotective, and stress-reducing effects. It reduces cortisol levels in the bloodstream and can also lower blood sugar levels and prevent gastric ulcers (great to calm an upset stomach). Drink as a tea or take by tincture, powder, or capsules. As always, follow the recommendations on the packaging.

Safety precautions for Holy basil (tulsi):

- Avoid if trying to get pregnant, when pregnant, or breastfeeding/lactating
- Contraindicated in patients with hypoglycemia

### Fish Oil

In addition to being a powerful anti-inflammatory, fish oil can aid in reducing stress and gut repair, and is particularly useful for brain health—60% of our brain is made up of DHA fat, so restoring those can help with cognitive function overall.

### A Good B Complex

B vitamins are essential ingredients for the production of your adrenal hormones—they are critical for relieving stress (your "Calgon, take me away" remedy in vitamin form), and particularly effective at combating fatigue and strengthening endurance. They, along with other nutrients, are important to biochemical processes occurring in your body 24/7 to keep it functioning optimally, including one called methylation. Methylation is a complex process of toxin removal and balance in the body. About 40% of the population has a genetic variation that hinders this process and they may need to take a methylated version of Vitamin B. It never hurts to default to this if you don't know for sure, but a simple genetic test can tell you if you have this variation.

## Vitamin C

Vitamin C is an essential cofactor in the production of adrenal hormones and supports the immune system. Studies show that it influences cortisol, inducing an anti-inflammatory response to prolonged exercise and extended stress.[65]

### RECIPE: COOL, CALM, & COLLECTED SMOOTHIE

The key to making a great-tasting and body-loving smoothie is including ingredients that not only taste delicious but that will satisfy you until your next meal. Smoothies are a great medium for getting a packed punch of nutrients. Note that this recipe is specifically tailored to stress reduction with the addition of ashwagandha. Swap this out for other superfoods like acai powder or turmeric for an antioxidant and/or anti-inflammatory boost.

**Ingredients**

4 to 6 ounces coconut milk

½ cup of frozen organic blueberries

1-2 cups of dark leafy greens

1-2 tablespoons of protein powder

1 teaspoon ashwagandha powder

1 tablespoon coconut oil—if you don't like the pebble-like texture, heat it gently to melt it before adding to your smoothie

½ cup ice (optional)

**Method**

Blend and enjoy. Tweak this recipe based on the flavors and consistency you like. For example, if you like a thicker smoothie, add in more ice cubes. Add more coconut milk or some water if you want it more liquid.

**Hormonious Tip:** Coconut oil provides a dose of healthy fat that will keep you sated. Well-known for its antioxidant and anti-viral properties, coconut oil has been shown to have anti-stress effects in animal studies.[66] Its functional benefits will make a great addition to your diet. I expand on the benefits of coconut oil in Chapter 6.

### *Be Creative with Adds and Swaps:*

- Coconut milk can be swapped out for other non-dairy milk alternatives:
  - o Almond
  - o Cashew
  - o Hazelnut
  - o Hemp seed
  - o Quinoa
  - o Rice

Experiment with 100% unsweetened juices, too, by using them as the base liquid or combining with the non-dairy liquid.

- Swap out blueberries for:
  - o Frozen acai (unsweetened)
  - o Frozen banana (remove peel and slice in chunks prior to freezing)
  - o Mango
  - o Pineapple
  - o Raspberries, blackberries, or strawberries

- Vegetables come in a variety of forms—get creative!
  - o Avocado
  - o Beets
  - o Cucumber
  - o Dark leafy greens (kale, spinach, etc.)
  - o Mint leaves

- Protein can be in the form of protein powder or a nut butter such as almond, walnut or cashew butter (one to two tablespoons), or whey powder (if you tolerate it)

- For extra crunch, add a tablespoon of almonds or walnuts

**Hormonious Tip:** L-glutathione is the master antioxidant. It is present in all cells and helps to maintain cell integrity. It plays a crucial role in immune function, detoxification and protection against oxidative stress. The best source is organic, grass-fed, non-denatured whey protein powder. Whey does not contain casein (a protein in dairy that many people cannot digest).

- Ashwagandha is used in this recipe for its stress-reducing powers. Swap this out for other superfood add-ins:

  o **Acai berries** pack a tremendous antioxidant punch. Purchase in the frozen fruit section of your supermarket and blend along with other berries.

  o **Bee pollen**, one of my favorites, is loaded with protein, vitamins, minerals, and antioxidants.

  o **Cacao nibs**, another favorite, are the inside meat of the cocoa bean—chocolate in its purest form! They are nutty and slightly bitter and contain antioxidants and minerals. They also add crunchy texture and marry well with nut butters or frozen blended banana.

  o **Cinnamon**—use ½ teaspoon for blood sugar balancing. Cinnamon manages cholesterol levels, too.

  o **Flax**, **chia**, or **hemp seeds**

- Flax seeds are high in fiber and contain anti-inflammatory omega-3 fatty acids, such as ALA (Alpha-linolenic acid). Flax seeds also contain lignans, which have estrogenic properties. I recommend them for post-menopausal women as one possible alternative to hormone-replacement therapy. To benefit from this effect, add one to two tablespoons of flax meal or flax oil daily into your smoothie.

- Chia seeds are high in fiber, protein, and omega-3s.

- Hemp seeds are known for their protein plus their perfect balance of omega-3s and omega-6s.

  o **Maca** is known not only for its stress-reducing influence but also for increasing energy. Its reputation as having a libido-boosting effect is sort of a turn-on. Maca has recently gained in popularity due to its ability to balance hormones. Some say it can help to reverse hypothyroidism.[67]

  o **Organic Super Greens** made by Paleo Valley is a powder and the perfect add-in if you are not a vegetable eater. Nutrient-dense, gluten-free, and highly absorbable. A no-brainer.

  o **Spirulina** has an earthy flavor and is a celebrated superfood with several assets: It contains protein, omega-3s, phytonutrients, and antioxidants, with the added bonus of chelating (or binding) heavy metals and removing them from the body.

# CHAPTER 4

# EXHAUSTED STATE OF MIND

*"Improper breathing is a common cause of ill health. If I had to limit my advice on healthier living to just one tip, it would be simply to learn how to breathe correctly ..., to spend time working on your breath and bringing more oxygen into your body and into your cells. There is no single more powerful—or more simple—daily practice to further your health and well-being than breathwork."*
—*Andrew Weil, M.D.*

**After my first son** was born, I did not want to go back to work. Wait, let me restart. Before my first son was born, I had no idea what to expect. I believed that two weeks off would be plenty of maternity leave before returning to the grind of practicing law. If you had a baby and thought you knew what it would be like and exactly how you would feel afterwards about work and life and parenting in general, you probably know what I'm talking about here. Suffice it to say, I was way off. The second he was born and my hormones took hold, I was off to a whole different set of races. Figuring out how to live on little sleep was something I'd never encountered before. My all-nighters from college days were not helpful or instructive, and did not prepare my body for coping with this reality.

Recognizing how challenged I was in performing my day job raised the concept of the need for sleep to the highest level of importance. My first new-mother idea was to find another job where I could get at least one day off. I found that job at a large law firm in Chicago. My part-time job meant I only had to bill 40 hours per week. (To a lawyer, 40 hours is "part-time.") This was a much lighter schedule than I had before and helped to some extent with balancing work, a new baby, and extra time off to sleep and recover.

Having worked in the field of law, I feel a sort of kinship to my fellow attorneys. After all, I understand what is expected, particularly at large law firms. The requirement for billing hours is incredibly stressful, leaving little time for anything else resembling a normal life. Years after I left the practice of law and began carving out my profession in women's health, I shared my new digs with a fellow attorney. He referred a colleague to my doorstep, and she became a client whose particular challenge (like mine so many years before) was total exhaustion.

Jill was 47 and working (fighting) to be partner in a boutique firm in the city. She was clocking in at 60 to 70 hours of work per week, but at the time that she started seeing me, her hours were dropping and she was taking time off for periodic "colds." In other words, she found herself getting so exhausted in the middle of the afternoon that she would literally have to take a nap at her desk and set an alarm so that she could get back to work 20 minutes later. In true *burning the candle at both ends* form, Jill had to take her work home with her, tending to it after she spent time with her boys and husband, feeding them dinner, and setting them up for the next day. Luckily for Jill, her husband was an asset and supported her in the household, allowing Jill that space to get her work done.

But her metaphorical brick house was starting to crumble. Jill was so exhausted that by the time the weekend came around, she was sleeping in the afternoons, which began to throw off her nighttime sleep. Once this started happening, her sleep schedule during the week was disrupted. She was either having difficulty falling asleep or she would find herself waking up in the middle of the night. This pattern was taking a toll on her, her work, and her family. She knew she needed help but wasn't quite sure how to get her life and sleep back. She did not like to work out and her diet was meh. I really liked Jill and we connected immediately, but I knew this was not going to be easy. I had my work cut out for me.

The piece that I knew I had in my favor was lab testing, as it would shed light on what was really going on with Jill. #TestDont-Guess has become one of my favorite hashtags not only because of the obvious—i.e., results in black and white are more meaningful than random guesswork—but because for some people (like Jill) objective results are motivating. The key for Jill to make changes and reverse the health-destroying situation she had unwittingly created was for her to see in facts and figures what was happening in her body, why she was so exhausted, and how her afternoon sleep sessions on the weekend made it impossible for her circadian rhythm to find its, well...rhythm.

Because Jill's main complaint was exhaustion and sleep deprivation, we only used two lab tests: one to measure her cortisol output and sex hormone levels, and the other to measure oxidative stress. My instinct was correct. I showed Jill that her cortisol levels were dropping severely in the afternoon along with an uptick of cortisol in the evening. These results correlated with Jill's description of her energy levels and fatigue. The result for the oxidative stress was only slightly out of range so I was less concerned about that, but I knew that the changes Jill would make would help the rise in oxidation in her body go in the other direction. She could finally see that the path she was on was going nowhere good, and that for her to feel better, she'd need to make changes.

While we tweaked some of Jill's eating habits (buh-bye, afternoon coffee and granola bars; hello, healthy fats, vibrant greens, and knockout proteins), the key piece for Jill was to change her schedule. Jill simply could not sustain the way she was working and living without an inevitable, possibly cataclysmic fallout. I first encouraged Jill to carve out time every day, a minimum of 20 minutes, to be used towards exercise, and 10 minutes to be used towards getting quiet and calm. Creating restorative space for quiet, meditation, or implementing simple breathing techniques is essential to rebalancing a body that is off kilter, especially like Jill's was.

Because Jill was already exhausted, however, we did not implement the changes in one fell swoop. Jill started out slowly by using her exercise time for walking. She was so tired, that when she began this new exercise journey, she could only manage walking around her neighborhood block. It took several weeks before she was able to increase her distance, which was fine. You need to start where you are. After she got used to walking, I encouraged her to go a little further every day, until she felt comfortable walking for a minimum of 20 minutes at a time. Eventually, she achieved 30 minutes. Walking, along with the restorative piece, were the building blocks for Jill to re-stabilize and reset her circadian rhythm. She was slowly starting to see how her (over)work ethic had taken a toll on her body, and her need to take care of it with nurturing time off was key to her healing process. We also eliminated the afternoon naps as these were disrupting her sleep-wake cycle and concentrated our focus on finding a way to balance her work with stress-reducing, as well as joy-lifting, activities.

The changes that Jill made were necessary to her ability to function. Along with the food and lifestyle changes Jill embraced, she also revamped the way she was working. She simply could not continue at the pace she was going without a serious breakdown. Instead, she created clear boundaries between her work life and home life: shutting off her cell phone when she came home from work; closing her computer down before dinner; and putting away work papers that could be dealt with the next day. As she made these changes, her sleep improved, and she slowly saw a return of energy. She was also spending quality time with her husband and was more engaged and present with her kids. She developed that internal compass and created an awareness muscle.

Because of the nature of Jill's work and her responsibilities to her family, she is still required to work extra sometimes. The difference now is that she has built into her life energetic reserves. Like a bank account, her weekend walks in the park, yoga workouts, vacations with her family, shutting work off at home, and breathing sessions all build up those energy savings. You see, for Jill it was not just about removing gluten, although Jill felt better without that, too. It was a full-on examination of how she was living her life and how her work was literally taking her down. Her willingness to honestly assess and then restructure her life meant that she could re-engage as she felt better. Caveat—Jill still has long, hard days. It just means her need for recovery needs to be honored, too, and thanks to her internal compass, she always finds time to refill her energy tank.

I understand what it means to work for hours and hours, and many people have to do this to pay bills and plan for the future, but exhausting the body's reserves in order to go-go-go every second for weeks on end will compromise your health. I guarantee it. Bodies are not designed for the kinds of demands we so often place on them, but by balancing your schedule and your lifestyle (that is, removing or revising what isn't working and doing more to replenish vitality), you really can restore your body to a state of dynamic health.

## Symptoms of poor sleep and low energy:

If you are low on energy and not sleeping well, you probably already know it. What you might not recognize are the many symptoms that can come from a chronic state of sleep deprivation and low energy. Do you experience any of the following?

- A need for coffee or stimulants in order to function
- An inability to handle stress
- Anxiety
- Brain fog
- Craving particular foods such as salt or sweet (this means you could be feeling weak and dizzy or experiencing drowsiness)
- Depression
- Dizziness when standing from a sitting or lying position
- Fatigue, insomnia, sleeplessness, exhaustion, lethargy, malaise
- Feeling rundown or overwhelmed
- Gaining weight around your middle
- Getting a second wind late at night, causing a "wired but tired" feeling that makes it difficult to fall asleep
- Having poor immunity where you catch everything that's going around
- Headaches and nausea, which can accompany a chronic lack of energy (typically, blood sugar balance is in the picture)
- Inability to recover from exercise
- Low sex drive, sadness, or feeling blah
- Memory issues
- Shakiness or irritability when you get overly hungry or skip meals
- Trouble waking up or not feeling refreshed when you do

- Waking in the middle of the night with a pounding heart

## Less obvious signs of sleep deprivation and low energy:

- Acne, rosacea
- Allergies
- Anxiety, emotional fragility
- Excessive weight gain or resistant weight loss
- Hypertension, cholesterol problems
- Indigestion, bloating
- Inflammation, pain, asthma
- PMS, irregular cycles

Do any of these symptoms resonate with you? If so, which ones? Add them to your Functional Timeline Plus if they aren't there already.

## THE SCIENCE BEHIND SLEEP DEPRIVATION AND LOW ENERGY

In general, we need approximately seven to eight hours of sleep each night for repair and recovery. If you're getting less than that, you may be experiencing cognitive deficits and perhaps having trouble performing your work and activities productively. Getting fewer hours for even several nights in a row is akin to staying awake for 24 hours straight.

When someone has reached a place where they are too tired to function, this is known as an exhaustive state. In FM, we call this by the technical-sounding term HPA axis dysregulation (HPAD). In further FM speak, symptoms are often referred to as appearing upstream or resulting downstream from a particular cause. Think about the root cause of your symptoms, and how from a root cause a symptom can appear as "downstream" from that root cause. For example, sleep disruptions and low energy are downstream effects of cortisol dysregulation (as discussed in Chapter 3). Working backwards, or looking upstream to cortisol dysregulation, means considering what is contributing to or causing that imbalance in cortisol. In the case of sleep issues, the main hormone to discuss on the subject of sleep is melatonin.

## Melatonin

Do you have a hard time falling asleep at night? Do you wake up in the middle of the night?

Either way, melatonin *and* cortisol are both at play.

Melatonin is a hormone produced in both your pineal gland (located in your brain) and your gut, where the majority, approximately 75%, is produced.[68] An unhappy gut can equal unhappy sleep. Melatonin affects the quality and duration of sleep and regulates the body's circadian rhythm. Humans follow a diurnal (opposite of nocturnal; think owls) pattern, so you are awake during the day (thank you, cortisol!) and require sleep at night to repair, rebuild, and detoxify your body plus give a rest to your adrenal glands. If cortisol is elevated at night, it can depress melatonin secretion, which interferes with the sleep/wake cycle. So, if you're having a hard time going to sleep at night, your cortisol levels may be higher than what they should be. Melatonin stores also decrease with aging, but there are ways to increase this hormone (see Fix Its at the end of this chapter).

> **Hormonious Tip:** Sleep deprivation impacts the body in other ways, too. Staying up late or working late shifts can put undue stress on the adrenal glands, hormones, blood sugar levels, and detox pathways and organs. Recall the concept of metabolic chaos, and the cascade effect on other systems when one system is imbalanced.

**Hormonious Tip:** Melatonin is very light-sensitive. The pineal gland senses light through your eyes, and this affects melatonin production. When traveling to destinations with a time change, the recommendation is to acclimate your body's circadian rhythm by following the local time, so even if it's 7:00 a.m. locally but your body thinks it's evening time, your shift and acceptance of the daylight will help your body's hormone production (i.e., cortisol) and nighttime melatonin adjust accordingly, even though it may take a period of days for that adjustment to settle. And because melatonin is sensitive to light, anything that you can do in the evening to reduce this factor will help support your body's natural impulse to produce this sleep-inducing hormone.

## YOUR LIVER + CHINESE MEDICINE

Do you wake up between 2 and 3 a.m.? One possible explanation for waking up in the middle of the night is a congested liver. It could be working overtime. Did you drink alcohol? Overeat? Did you eat food late in the evening? According to Chinese medicine, the period between 11 p.m. and 3 a.m. is when the liver is repairing. If it's been overburdened, it might let you know by waking you up. Sort of a reminder to "pay attention" to what you're demanding of it. While conventional medicine doesn't recognize the concept of a "congested liver" (for example, according to a Chinese medicine doctor, you may have normal liver enzymes yet still suffer from a sluggish liver), the liver's role in detoxification may be impaired if it can't keep pace with the amount of toxins coming at it. This can contribute to specific problems such as when a sluggish liver can't aid in the conversion of thyroid hormone or efficiently clear excess estrogen (more information on this in the following pages and in Chapter 5).

While decreased melatonin can lead to sleep disturbances, there may be other contributing factors in the mix such as blood sugar imbalance or nutrient deficiencies. If you sometimes wake up in the middle of the night because you're feeling hungry, actually due to low blood sugar, these may be the culprits. Low magnesium levels and lack of sufficient Vitamin B can also be contributing factors to poor sleep. Moving upstream, if you're not absorbing these nutrients (even though you may be eating foods or taking supplements), consider your digestive health.

> **Hormonious Tip:** These are some of the things that inhibit the production of melatonin:
>
> - **Caffeine, alcohol consumption, and steroid drugs.** A recent study found that consumption of caffeine three hours before bedtime induced a 40-minute delay of the circadian melatonin rhythm.[69] Simply put, caffeine can interfere with sleep. Some people have a genetic variant that slows the metabolism of caffeine in their systems. Those slow metabolizers who drink coffee early in the afternoon may have difficulty with their sleep.
> - **NSAIDs** (like Ibuprofen) **are melatonin inhibitors.** Zyflamend may be an appropriate alternative—it contains herbs to help address occasional pain.
> - **Large doses of B12.** Your B12 vitamin should be taken in the morning, or it may be keeping you up at night.

## ADRENAL GLANDS AND THE HPA AXIS

You may be familiar with the concept of "adrenal fatigue," a condition supposedly characterized by chronic tiredness or exhaustion due to the malfunction of or poor functioning of the adrenal glands. Trendy as it may be to suspect this condition, the truth is that unless the adrenal glands are in a state of disease, such as Addison's disease, exhaustion is likely to be a problem related to more than just the adrenal glands. Instead, I prefer to look at how well the entire hypothalamic/pituitary/adrenal axis is functioning in response to stress, since these three endocrine glands all work together to govern your body's stress response. Specifically, how well is the brain communicating with the HPA axis, and how well is the body handling the cascade of interrelated hormones produced in response to stress? Recall in Chapter 3 when I told you about how the hormone cortisol is upregulated during periods of stress, and that during periods of chronic stress, cortisol can be constantly produced and circulated, as directed by the brain and various feedback mechanisms. The body does this because its priority is to save you from that "bear in the woods." However, as you have already learned, the body has limited resources and simply isn't designed to handle continual exposure to an overabundance of stress.

Over time, fighting that bear constantly, day in and day out (or in more conventional terms: working from morning to night in an extremely demanding environment, fighting the constant headache of traffic, caring for the emotional and financial demands of children or elderly parents, and all other possible stresses you may be experiencing simultaneously in your life) can tip the body into a state of exhaustion, especially for those who don't have the metabolic reserves to stand up to those constant stresses. Fatigue is a downstream effect of chronic stress. The body is losing its ability to adjust and adapt, and its resources are being spent. It's a bigger-picture scenario than the functioning of the adrenals in isolation.

In order to determine how to fix your exhaustion, you have to consider how you got here in the first place. Why are you exhausted? And what can you do about it? The Fix Its at the end of this chapter can support you as you take steps to return your system to a functioning equilibrium. You might also want to review Chapter 2, if the stresses in your life loom large. The important thing is to take steps to replenish your body with the energy and resources it requires so that it can return to allostasis, and all the parts of your energy-producing system (including your adrenals) can start working the way they are supposed to again.

## THYROID HORMONES AND ENERGY

Your thyroid, located in front of your trachea at the base of your throat, has a huge impact on overall health and metabolism, serving as the metabolic regulator for every cell in your body. It secretes only two hormones, T3 (triiodothyronine) and T4 (thyroxine). T3 and T4 regulate your body's temperature, metabolism, and heart rate. The amount of thyroid hormone secreted is controlled by another hormone, called thyroid stimulating hormone (TSH), which is released from the pituitary gland in your brain. The pituitary gland ensures that the right amount of hormone is produced by the thyroid.

An overactive thyroid, known as **hyperthyroid**, means that too much T3 and T4 are produced and there's an abundance of energy. Symptoms like insomnia, nervousness, hair loss, racing heart, hot flashes (also influenced by falling estrogen), and weight loss are common to hyperthyroidism. However, in the case of an underactive thyroid, **hypothyroid**, where the gland is not producing enough T3 and T4, metabolism slows and there is a loss of energy. Symptoms can be weight gain, tiredness, difficulties concentrating or slowed thinking, and constipation. Hypothyroidism can also impact sleep, as there's a complete slowdown in all metabolic processes, throwing off the whole system.

One of the tricky things doctors face when diagnosing thyroid problems is that the thyroid can present as normal in thyroid tests but be functioning abnormally. There are a lot of different things that could potentially impact the thyroid, many of which may be outside the thyroid gland. For example:

- Autoimmunity
- Electromagnetic fields[70]

- Environmental toxins[71]

- Gut inflammation

- HPA axis dysfunction

- Impaired detoxification

- Infections

- Nutrient deficiencies

- Oxidative stress

- Radiation

- Stress

Standard medical treatment for the thyroid tends to focus exclusively on the thyroid gland; e.g. thyroid hormone replacement, anti-thyroid medication, radioactive iodine therapy, and/or thyroid surgery. These therapies may, of course, be appropriate. However, addressing the underlying causes of thyroid dysfunction is essential to zeroing in on the treatment that will actually solve the problem (the basis of the FM paradigm).

Typically, there is no single cause of thyroid hormone dysregulation, but several. This is why restoring balance to the body is so important. Instead of looking at one organ and pointing the finger at it, restore general health and the thyroid is often able to repair itself. How cool is that?!

Nevertheless, if you are exhausted during the day and having difficulty sleeping at night, please have your thyroid hormone levels checked. An underactive thyroid can be caused by an iodine deficiency, or Hashimoto's thyroiditis, an autoimmune condition in which the thyroid is being attacked by the immune system. There may be a genetic component, and other medications can also be a contributing factor to a slowed-down metabolism. If everything looks fine, consider visiting an FM practitioner for more in-depth testing and/or work on integrating the Fix Its at the end of this chapter into your daily routine.

# THE LINK BETWEEN ENERGY AND CARBS

Carbs have become controversial, which is actually kind of strange, considering that most foods contain at least some (only meat and fat are carb-free). Detractors say they cause everything from low energy to obesity, but the truth is a bit more complicated.

Carbs are a structural component of cell membranes and a source of fiber. They provide energy to the body, so why do they also sometimes seem to drain it? The supposed energy spikes and crashes we get from carbs are really about blood sugar dysregulation, not the blanket effect of carbohydrates. The body does not treat all carbs the same. Some carbs do raise blood sugar, especially in large amounts, which causes an answering rise in insulin.[72] Others are unlikely to cause this problem. For example, phytonutrient-rich vegetables and dark leafy greens contain carbs, but these foods provide your cells with the nutrient-rich energy, vitamins, and minerals your body requires to operate efficiently and at peak performance. When these energy-driving foods are absent, your cells are missing out on important energy-producing effects.

Then you've got refined foods heavy with sugar and white flour, highly devoid of the nutrients your cells crave. These also contain carbs, but unlike vegetables, these carbs are more likely to cause an extreme rise in blood sugar, followed by an extreme rise in insulin, which causes an extreme drop in blood sugar, which causes an extreme drop in energy. So many extremes! No wonder you're tired.

These energy-sucking foods—the ones many people typically grab in the morning or eat as a snack during the day, like bagels, muffins, sugary cereals, donuts, candy bars, granola bars, cookies, cakes, and bread—are on the Most Wanted list for energy-killers, too. Do you notice a drop in energy after downing a plateful of pancakes drenched in syrup? I know I do.

The solution is pretty simple, though—if you have issues with low energy, get the refined carbs out of your diet. That alone might solve your problem. Think about that the next time you are eyeing the vending machine or the breakfast menu, and let your knowledge inform your decisions about what to eat.

> **Hormonious A-ha!:** When fatigue is part of your health struggle equation, low levels of magnesium, iron, or B12 are at the top of the culprit list. Magnesium levels can be checked with your doctor. In the case of iron, simply eating more red meat won't necessarily solve your problem. Some people eat foods rich in iron but still have low ferritin levels (a measure of iron stores). If this is the case for you, I recommend considering the state of your stomach acid levels. Low stomach acid means that you are not properly breaking down iron and B12. See Chapter 2's Fix It section for DIY instructions on evaluating your stomach acid levels. If you don't feel comfortable doing a self-assessment, ask your FM practitioner about testing your stomach acid, B12, and ferritin levels (the FM range for ferritin is 90-110 ng/mL). Looking for root causes requires you to think strategically, and again, upstream: the health of your digestive tract, possible malabsorption, and poor diet can also be considered. Knowing your exact deficiencies can help you take targeted steps to repair them, either through foods or supplements.

## FIX IT

Get calm, be present, and know that there is a road out of this exhausted and low-energy state. Be kind to yourself and envision the life you will have when you recover. Don't ever lose sight of this. Step by step is the way forward.

## What to Do

### Sleep-Inducing Tips

If you are having difficulties falling asleep, or waking up in the middle of the night, or if your sleep is not restorative and you are not waking up refreshed, it's time to renovate your sleep habits and create a routine for sound sleep; a.k.a., practice better sleep hygiene. Preparing your body for bed can help boost the natural production of melatonin and cue your cortisol to chill out until morning. Good habits can retrain your circadian rhythm.

If you find that after practicing the following strategies, you are still having trouble sleeping, or waking up in the middle of the night, consider looking upstream for other contributing factors, such as those suggested above and in previous chapters. Your sleep hygiene protocol should include the following:

### *Exercise during the day to sleep better at night.*[73, 74,]

If you are not doing any form of exercise whatsoever, I encourage you to start walking. If Jill can do it, so can you. Start slowly by walking around your neighborhood block. If you live in an apartment building, you can walk the floors and use the stairs (you get bonus points for using the stairs!). Additional bonus points if you can walk in a park, forest preserve, or any outdoor setting with trees, grass, and nature. (You will find more examples of exercise in Chapter 5.)

### *Finish eating three hours before you go to sleep.*

Optimal digestion occurs through the magic of gravity while you're sitting upright. It's stressful on the body and the liver to digest food when you are horizontal, which can be a cause for waking you in the middle of the night.

### *Write out your worries.*

In many cases, your sleep problems are an outgrowth of your state of mind. Perhaps you are unable to turn your mind off, or the day's stresses have seeped into your nighttime routine. To offset this happening, find structured time during the week or on the weekend to do some freestyle writing. Writing is one of the most cathartic methods to unwind from the grip of stress that is interfering with your need to sleep. It also clears the mind and re-trains its focus. It doesn't matter what you write about, but spending time venting on paper with a pen or on a computer will not only provide a space for you to unleash your frustrations, worries, or concerns, but may also provide an opportunity for you to find insight or solutions to some of the issues that are keeping you up at night. This is a highly recommended tool to use on your journey towards transformation.

- Purchase a lined notepad or open up a new document and let loose. Another option is to incorporate "morning writing pages."[75] Set your alarm to an hour before you typically wake up. Without getting out of bed, or performing any of your morning activities, write for three straight pages. Again, it doesn't matter what you write about. What might happen, however, is that you'll start writing about how you got here, what's happening now, and how you want to change it. This may be the key to your next steps. Get to writing. And try to do it every morning. See how this activity can be life-changing. You're welcome.

- Caveat: don't do this just prior to going to sleep, unless doing so is helpful. It could be an agitating process and make going to sleep more difficult. If this is the case, find a time during the day to get your vent-writing done.

- If you have attempted this recommendation and simply do not like to write, consider expressing (read: venting, relieving, discharging) yourself through other creative outlets. Expressing creativity to relieve sadness or frustration is underrated in our culture. Painting with watercolors, acrylics, or even oil-based paints on a blank canvas can help to unleash some of the thoughts that may be getting in your way. Finding activities that captivate your attention means you are not only able to be present in that activity but that those niggling thoughts are less of a distraction. The more often you engage your mind and brain in this kind of creative nourishment, the greater the distance you will develop from those negative thoughts. Then, sleep may come easier. Choose an activity to set your creativity free and that can, in the process, unload some baggage. Don't think you're creative? No problem. Try an adult coloring book or use the app Lake for coloring in pre-drawn designs.

### Get touched.

Touch is a healing commodity and therapeutic for a body that is exhausted. When possible, arrange for a massage in the evening hours that will prepare your body for rest and soothe tension and sore muscles away. Professional hugging is a real thing. In need of a cuddle? Check out cuddlist.com for a restorative embrace.

### Take a hot bath.

Ready a hot bath and add in two cups of Epsom salt (magnesium sulfate will be absorbed into the skin) for its relaxing properties. The heat of the water will loosen up tight muscles, and the steam will give your body an opportunity to sweat and detoxify. Add eight drops of lavender oil, as this essential oil is known for reducing cortisol. If you don't have time for a bath, purchase a diffuser so that you can get the benefits of lavender upon inhalation.[76]

### Zen your bedroom.

Make your bed a welcome, awesome, beautiful, peaceful, zen-like space. Clean, quality sheets will set the tone. Clear away clutter and store non-essentials out of sight. Keep your nightstand tidy and your room neat so that if I were to come over for a visit, you'd be proud to show me your bedroom. How old is your mattress? If your answer is "very," consider replacing it. After all, you spend a third of your life sleeping in bed. Make it warm, welcoming, and inviting to you.

### Dim it.

Install dimmer switches in your bedroom and other rooms you spend time in the evening so that as you're readying yourself for bed, you can taper down the light to support melatonin production. If you can't install dimmers, consider purchasing blue light-blocking glasses to use at night to block out artificial light.

### Reserve it.

Consider your bed for purposes of sleep and sex only.

### Get rid of screens.

Keep screens out of your bedroom. If watching TV until you fall asleep has become a habit, unplug (or better yet, remove) your television from the bedroom. Let's undo this one for good. Maybe there's another location in your home that could use this set. Remove all other electronics from your bedroom (especially your smartphone). Although this is a controversial notion, there is evidence to suggest that electromagnetic fields (EMFs) adversely affect melatonin production.[77] If you are not willing to move your phone out of your room, then turn it to airplane mode to eliminate the EMFs or off altogether to eliminate exposure to blue light. Finally, even if you moved the TV out and keep your computer elsewhere, avoid using these devices at least one to two hours before bedtime. They are stimulating to the brain, making it harder to fall asleep and impairing the body's ability to calm down and keep the nervous system in a state of sympathetic dominance. Using blue light blocking glasses while on these devices can minimize the impact on melatonin production.

### Read...maybe.

If reading does not interfere with your falling asleep, then by all means, keep doing it. However, if your reading material is thought-provoking or stimulating, you may want to save it for daytime reading.

### Get comfy.

Consider using a body pillow between your knees to support your spine if you are a stomach or side sleeper. Replace pillows that are uncomfortable and extremely worn.

*Keep your room cool and dark.*

Our body temperature drops at night and prefers a lower temperature, ranging optimally between 60 to 67 degrees. The darker, the cooler, the better—light inhibits melatonin production and you'll be supporting your body's production by following this simple tip.

*Turn in early.*

Aim to be in bed by 10:00 p.m., preferably not later than 10:30. Hold fast to this window until you can re-establish a stable sleep routine. It may be difficult at first, but you are retraining your body and getting back into sync with your natural circadian rhythm, so stay with it.

*Relax.*

Try this relaxation-inducing nightly routine: Find a comfortable position, either on a cushion, in a chair, or reclining in bed. If on a cushion, you can sit with your legs crossed, or stretched out in front of you. Relax your face, muscles, and all your body parts. Close your eyes and inhale. Hold for several seconds, then exhale. Do this several more times, all the while concentrating on the sounds your breath is making inside of your body. Feel your lungs filling and expanding on each inhale and releasing on each exhale. Breathe in deeply, so that your belly is expanding. Exhale all of the air out. Next, concentrate on each body part, starting with your toes, stretching them in all directions, and then relax them. Move up to the ankles and move them in all directions. Stretch and relax them. Do this to each successive body part moving up your body. Knees, hips, pelvis, buttocks, fingers, hands, wrists, elbows, shoulders, neck. Aim to spend 10 to 20 minutes doing this until you are in a complete zone of calm. It is natural that various thoughts will pass through. Let them enter and exit or do what they will. Refrain from judgment or frustration. It's completely natural, and over time, these thoughts will impact you less and less and may become infrequent or stop altogether. The objective is to focus on your breath and your body, and to move into a state of calm and relaxation.

> **Hormonious Caution:** If you are following the sleep hygiene tips above and do not experience a notable difference within a period of two to four weeks, you may have a hidden stressor that requires further investigation. Food sensitivities, pathogens, or leaky gut can all be contributing to your sleep issues and lack of energy or a result of it—dysbiosis and pathogens become more stimulating at night and set off stress responses, thus interfering with your ability to sleep.

## Energy-Inducing Tips

Just getting better sleep will help increase energy, but there are some other ways to get the energy surging back into your day:

***Gentle exercise like walking or stretching is one of the surest ways to combat fatigue.***

If during the workday you find yourself wanting to nap or can't keep your eyes open, this is the time to take a walk outside, get fresh air, and do some stretching at your desk. While sitting with your back straight, bend your head down towards your chest and roll it to the right, making a big, sweet circle. Do the same to the left. Now stand, keeping your body erect, and reach both arms up towards the ceiling. Bring your left arm down and reach your right arm over your head in the direction towards your left hip. Bend at the hip in the same direction. Do the same on the other side. After you do this, clasp your hands behind your back and bend forward at the hip, keeping your shoulders down. If this stretch feels good, let your shoulders move with gravity towards your head. Next, twist your body slowly and gently, in both directions with your feet firmly in place. The last move is to stretch up on your toes if your shoes allow it (or remove them for this part), so that you're standing tippy-toe. This bit of stretching will provide a little energy boost and move you through your day.

### Monitor your blood sugar.

If you are suffering from exhaustion or lack of energy during the day, it will be worth your investment to monitor your blood sugar levels and take heed to what you are eating. Doing so is simple and fairly non-invasive. Purchase a glucometer on Amazon, along with test strips and lancets. The general ideal range is 80-90 mg/dL (4.2-5.0 mmol/L), though this can vary from person to person. The easiest way to keep track of your blood sugar is with an app. There are several: Glucose - Blood Sugar Tracker, Glucose Buddy, or Blood Sugar Monitor will help you stay organized. Check your blood sugar before breakfast, lunch, and dinner and before bed for several days. Recheck it after you begin to modify your diet and reduce refined carbs. I'll cover the foods to avoid so that blood sugar balance can be maintained.

> **Hormonious Tip:** Do not skip meals. Honor your body's need for a steady stream of energy and avoid the pitfalls that accompany a plunge in your blood sugar. Skipping meals disrupts blood sugar levels and slows your metabolic rate. This will mess with your energy levels, throwing off your cortisol and leaving you exhausted.

### Eat foods that are energetic and that will translate in your body as energy.

The process of reclaiming your energy starts with eating foods that fuel your body's cells.

- The most energy-producing foods are dark leafy greens and vegetables. Add these into every meal. Purchase a container of organic mixed greens or arugula that can be added by the handful to any meal you're eating. Today, many of these packaged greens are pre-washed. Easy!

- Eat pastured eggs, grass-fed meats or pasture-raised poultry, and wild-caught fish.

- Balance out your fiber-rich carbs and proteins with healthy fats like avocados, olives, and coconut oil. They will provide your body with additional stores of energy.

- Add in iron-rich foods to boost your iron stores. Sometimes fatigue is masked by an iron deficiency. Here are a few you can incorporate:
  - Asparagus
  - Beans
  - Bok choy
  - Clams
  - Cumin
  - Dark leafy greens
  - Eggs
  - Leeks
  - Lentils
  - Organ meats
  - Oysters
  - Parsley
  - Poultry
  - Red meats
  - Shellfish
  - Turmeric

## WHAT NOT TO EAT

***Avoid high-glycemic foods.***
These not only raise blood sugar but can impact melatonin as well.

- Eliminate all grains (including whole grain and sprouted breads), sugars, and fruit juices. Do this for a period of at least 30 days until your blood sugar is in a good balance.

- Avoid cereals, flours, rice, corn, and white potatoes. If this is too difficult for you, small portions of organic rice or quinoa can help through this transition. For best results, avoid the white stuff and corn for at least 30 days.

- Limit fruits to berries and other low-glycemic options. Once blood sugar is under control, a wider variety of fresh fruits and items like potatoes and rice may be added back in. Avoid dried or tinned fruits—they are loaded with sugar and bring your energy down.

- Reduce/eliminate caffeine, alcohol, and sugar and refined carbs, as these impact melatonin levels,[78] particularly since they are typically ingested at later hours of the day. To reduce your caffeine intake, see Chapter 5 in the Fix It section to learn how.

- If you have low blood pressure and experience dizziness upon standing, drink coconut water or add sea salt to your meals. This will raise blood pressure and combat fatigue.

## WHAT TO EAT / DRINK

***Eat protein before bed, as needed.***
If you are waking in the middle of the night and hungry, your blood sugar balance may be off. To counteract this, eat a small amount of protein that contains the amino acid tryptophan, a precursor to melatonin; for example, a slice of turkey, chunk of salmon, one tablespoon or two of pumpkin seeds, or pumpkin seed butter. Tryptophan helps to induce sleep, has a natural calming effect, and helps regulate blood sugar levels.

*Increase melatonin levels with these additional melatonin-rich foods.*

- Almonds
- Bananas
- Flax seed
- Goji berries
- Oranges
- Pineapple
- Raspberries
- Rice
- Sweet corn
- Tart cherries or cherry juice
- Tomatoes
- Walnuts

### Just say yes to fatty fish.

Healthy fats that promote energy also support sleep. A great source is wild-caught fatty fish such as Atlantic salmon.[79]

### Eat Vitamin D-rich foods.

Vitamin D is essential to sound health and sleep.[80] It's a fat-soluble nutrient that is actually a hormone! Vitamin D is responsible for a long list of bodily functions, including blood sugar regulation, bone development and maintenance, metabolism, cell growth and development, insulin secretion, and immune system function.

Here are foods that will boost your Vitamin D levels:

- Butter
- Eggs
- Herring

- Liver

- Mackerel

- Mushrooms

- Salmon

- Sardines, canned

- Shrimp

- Sunflower seeds

- Tuna

### Add weeds to your diet.

Purslane is a weed that contains melatonin and significant amounts of beta-carotene, Vitamin C, and antioxidants. It also has high levels of omega-3 fatty acids—five times higher than spinach. It grows best in hot regions such as the southern portion of the U.S. You may find it at farmers' markets in the summer—or you may find it growing in your yard or garden. Purslane makes a great addition to salads and smoothies.

### Drink hot tea.

Hot herbal teas that contain sleep-inducing herbs are perfect to add into your night-time regimen. Valerian root, chamomile, and lemon root are all great options to get you sleepy. (Avoid teas containing caffeine.)

## WHAT TO TAKE

### Supplement with magnesium.

Magnesium glycinate and magnesium citrate are available as capsules or in a powdered form that can be mixed with water prior to sleep. I highly recommend Calm magnesium powder by Natural Vitality. A spoonful mixed with water in the evening will get your body and brain ready to snooze. These forms are easily absorbed and can help prepare your body for sleep as well as increase your magnesium levels (these can be checked with a simple blood test at your doctor's office—many people are deficient). Magnesium glycinate is particularly known for easing anxiety, while magnesium citrate is also helpful for constipation. If you prefer to supplement with a capsule, 200-400mg is a recommended dose.

### Consider melatonin.

Melatonin is sometimes used to support your body's natural melatonin production. The time-released version is best if you tend to wake up in the middle of the night. Follow the instructions for dosages, with the supervision of your doctor, and consider this supplement as a stand-in until your system is back on track.

### Consider *phosphatidylserine* to lower cortisol.

Phosphatidylserine is an amino acid and fatty substance, a.k.a. phospholipid. It is produced by foods and by your body and is an important part of the cell membrane, supporting messaging and nerve impulse and improving brain function. While this supplement has been praised for its effects on the symptoms of Alzheimer's[81] disease, some practitioners recommend it for its usefulness in lowering cortisol[82] and help with insomnia. Soy lecithin delivers the highest amount of phosphatidylserine bang for your food buck (as does cow brain, but mad cow disease has made this a no-go choice), so pay attention to supplement ingredients and opt for soy-free options as needed. Other foods high in phosphatidylserine include:

- Organ meats such as kidneys, liver, and hearts
- Atlantic mackerel, herring, and cod
- White beans
- Chicken meat with skin (dark meat contains more than white)

### Defend against free radicals with CoQ10.

Also known as ubiquinone, coenzyme Q10 is known primarily for its antioxidant and anti-aging properties and considered an essential nutrient. It is necessary for producing cellular energy, as well as for defending against free radicals. It helps other enzymes perform their digestive function and increases the absorption of other essential nutrients. Other benefits of CoQ10 include supporting blood sugar regulation and helping to lower fatigue and boost stamina (Goodbye, exhaustion!). Your body naturally creates CoQ10 but declines as you reach middle age. Because CoQ10 is fat-soluble, absorption will be enhanced by taking it with foods that contain fat.

## RECIPE: ENERGIZE YOUR DAY SALAD

Here's a delicious lunch salad to energize you in the afternoon.

### Ingredients

Any mixed salad greens (dark and leafy like kale, spinach, or arugula, etc.)

One small tomato, diced

One small cucumber, chopped

One tablespoon chopped purple onion

Several Kalamata olives

¼ cup crumbled goat feta (if tolerated)

Two to three wild-caught sardines (if small, add more)

### Dressing

Drizzle extra virgin olive oil, lemon juice, salt, and pepper on top. Assemble and enjoy.

### *Be Creative with Adds and Swaps:*

- Chopped walnuts, slivered almonds, sunflower or pumpkin seeds are great options.

- Rotate greens by using romaine, rocket lettuce, or other available leaf lettuce.

- Swap out tomatoes and cucumbers for diced beets, artichoke hearts, or bell peppers.

- In place of feta, use ½ a diced avocado.

- If you don't like sardines, replace with hard-boiled egg, chicken, salmon, or other lean meat.

- In place of meats, add ¼ cannellini beans or other legume.

- Leftover baked, grilled, or sautéed veggies can also be swapped in.

This recipe provides a composition of fat, fiber, and protein, and a sample from which you can swap or add vegetables, nuts, and seeds.

# CHAPTER 5

# WHEN THE MOOD STRIKES

*"If you want to live a happy life, tie it to a goal, not to people or objects."*
—*Albert Einstein*

Mood drives much of our life experience. It can make or break your day, and it can make your efforts towards better health feel diminished. While everyone has moods, including ups and downs, highs and lows, a woman's unique physiology to procreate makes her the repository of more hormones and processes than a man has. She has the ability to create life, but that necessary hormonal complexity can also mean more health complexity in general, and more mood complexity specifically. From puberty to menstrual fluctuations to perimenopause and menopause (and pregnancy, for those who experience it), women are subject to the unpredictability of our physiology. You may move through some of these stages questioning your sanity, crying a lot, or feeling like your emotional ups and downs are unpredictable and uncontrollable. The first step to regaining control is to recognize the interplay and connection between sex hormones and neurotransmitters,[83] and I'm going to help you with that. But first, I want to tell you about Laura.

I met Laura at a talk I gave soon after I launched my business. I was excited to be sharing my newfound knowledge that food is medicine, and Laura appreciated one of my favorite recipes, Simplify Truffles (recipe to come later in this chapter). I had made a batch for my talk and gave them away at the end so attendees could make the connection between food, medicine, and a treat that was delicious and had health benefits—a method I have found works well for the food-obsessed, especially those of us with a sweet tooth.

About a year after that talk, Laura reached out to me wondering if I could help her. She is a single mom of one and works for a not-for-profit. She was 49 at the time we started working together, and she complained that she wasn't quite feeling herself the past several months. Specifically, she was noticing a change in her moods. She wasn't her cheerful, easygoing self and observed her behavior being irritable, cranky, and impatient. She reported that she felt a little blue and teary-eyed on occasions that didn't warrant tears.

She had been to her doctor and nothing unusual came out of that visit, although he advised her to keep in touch if her tears turned into something greater. Her gynecologist reported that she was probably experiencing perimenopausal symptoms due to her fluctuating hormones. He gave her general instructions to eat healthier, make sure she was getting enough sleep, and, of course, keep exercising. Both visits were disappointing for her. She was hoping for more insight into what was going on. She was still menstruating, but that was also a changing tide. Some months were spotty and others she was full-blown in it.

Laura wanted to feel better and she recalled my lecture and those tasty truffles. She wanted to see how I could help her make changes and whether that might help her peculiar and unsettling mood events. After reviewing her health history, I saw nothing glaring. She had had various UTIs (antibiotics alert) over the years, and had finalized her divorce from her husband of 17 years within months of our initial meeting. Caring for her aging parents also weighed on her. Fortunately, Laura had a tightknit family including three siblings who all shared the burden of overseeing her parents' needs. Her son was 17 and a senior in high school. He would be leaving for college come fall—another stressful and poignant mile-stone event for many parents.

Considering Laura's age, the stress of her divorce, her only child leaving the home shortly, and her aging parents, I could see how her story might be about significant changes happening, as well as an important transition for her. Her life was going through a revision, a rewrite of sorts, which can be both uncomfortable and scary—the perfect recipe for mood issues. She was obviously stressed, and as you may already suspect, mood issues are another issue down-stream of stress. Laura had reached that sweet spot age where the transition into menopause is no longer a theory learned in school. Rather, changes were manifesting on a physiological level.

Our lives are a collection of experiences. After evolving from childhood to adulthood and all that it entails, families develop, children are born, parents age, a loved one passes away, and so the world turns. Yet, it is in these transitions that people experience difficulty and are sometimes tested. Have you built up a foundation of resilience to weather these storms? Your physiology, genetics, and interaction with the environment are all variables.

For Laura, I recognized that she needed help reframing this transition into one of opportunity rather than crisis so that she could start to hone in on the cause of those moods and implement ways to tame them. In part, the protocol I created for Laura was based on implementing a series of lifestyle changes along with tweaks to her diet. Her sleep was erratic and she had become a bit of a homebody, spending little to no time with friends and giving up on her favorite hobbies of listening to live music and dancing.

Her preoccupation with managing her divorce, worry about her parents, and sadness that her child would be out of the house distracted and stifled her from doing or enjoying the things that she loved. Yet, she wasn't in the mood to listen to music or go dancing.

But this withdrawal was okay for her, temporarily. She needed this period of time to explore what her next chapter would be. Her moods were clues for her to assess her life, evaluate the road she was on, and decide whether she wanted to keep going or choose a different path. Sometimes, when someone needs space and time to adjust, it can seem stressful or feel like a strain, particularly when interactions and activities that brought you joy no longer seem to do so. This feeling may seem completely foreign to you. You know something is off but you can't put your finger on it, don't know why it's happening, and just can't seem to shake it off. While this is often due to the fear of change and the unknown, it is also a reflection of an inner compass that has been hijacked by the demands of life and is no longer functioning at peak performance.

But what if you could replace that strain with acceptance? In the Fix Its, I introduce one of my favorite mottos: "This Is Where I'm At." The idea behind these words is that it's okay to embrace yourself no matter where you are in your life right now or how you feel at that moment. Start by acknowledging that your life and body are experiencing a particular set of circumstances. This recognition can help to anchor you in time and clear your mind of the stress of trying to force some mindset about your current circumstances. What if, instead of feeling anxiety and dread, you let yourself feel a sense of possibility and anticipation for what's coming next? Ultimately, the idea is to surrender to this moment, while still putting one foot in front of the other. And yet, change doesn't have to be huge. It could be small. It could be manageably medium-sized. Even if the change you are experiencing is major due to your circumstances, your point of transition, and/or your ultimate desires, let that enliven and invigorate you. Take your time getting there, too. That is, allow yourself the gift of time to slow down to thoughtfully consider your next move(s).

In Laura's case, she was smack dab in the middle of a major evolution in her body, in her spousal relationship, and in her roles as both a mother and a daughter. Each aspect change was fraught with coinciding mood effects. This is not uncommon for women who hit their mid-40s. If it's happening to you, I encourage you to find the joy, expectation, and hope in your situation. Change is an opportunity, and considering whether your moods are an outgrowth of those circumstances can give you more insight into yourself, your situation, and your next direction. If the change is coming, you might as well make the best of it and honor your anxiety or sadness as you move from one phase to the next. With this in mind, I invite you to stay present, through every moment, every mood, and mood event, and dial into your awareness. Even small changes can be transformative, and any change could prompt you to do something new (something you've always wanted to do perhaps?) and also help you evaluate your entire life so far, including your relationships, health, and work satisfaction.

Laura's process to a more stable mood took a period of several months.

Keys to her success were spending time examining her next stage in life, preparing for her son's departure, upgrading her food choices, and joining a women's book club. She started meeting with friends on a weekly basis, and even joined a gym so that she could take a dance exercise class. She had to mourn the ending of her marriage to the man she thought she would live out the rest of her life with. These lifestyle upgrades and adjustments were not immediate. She added each one slowly as it felt right and made sense to her as she navigated back to her cheery self. In the case where you are troubled by moods, time and patience with yourself are your best allies.

**Hormonious Tip:** Remember to include big life events and transitions in your Functional Timeline Plus. Tracking these not only provides the broader context of your life experiences but can explain some of the fallout that may be happening as a result of them. Writing this out can be validating. Your experiences are your experiences! How you pass through them, learn from them, and grow is your process of building a greater resilience for the next possible big event. Your evolution through them is also an opportunity for strengthening your interior network and continuing to develop that internal compass of awareness, a close cousin to resilience.

## MOODY MUCH?

Moods are complex and ever-changing. We all have a right to feel a wide range of emotions—happiness, sadness, fear, joy, excitement, or boredom. This is part of what it means to be human. However, if your moods feel mostly uncomfortable or unsustainable, that's when you need an intervention. The term "mood swings" is defined as extreme or rapid changes in mood.

Ideally, you will spend a lot of time feeling good—light, calm, cheerful, hopeful, confident, intentional, etc. That is the goal. Most importantly, you should never feel hostage to your moods. (If you are experiencing manic highs and depressive lows, a psychologist can evaluate whether this is a condition that requires deeper support and professional treatment.)

Let's take a look at how you are feeling right now, assess your dominant mood in the last few months, and start the process to eke out the root cause. For our purposes, beyond the situations you may be able to work out with friends or a therapist, mood changes are often triggered by, or worsened by, the hormonal imbalance that comes with perimenopause or hormonal imbalances from other causes. High rates of depression during menopause are not uncommon.[84] Further, research discovered that the brain protein MAO-A (enzyme monoamine oxidase A), linked to depression, is more abundant in perimenopausal women than younger women or women who have reached menopause.[85] Is this happening to you?

Are you experiencing any of these symptoms?

- Anxiety
- Anxiousness, nervousness
- Binge or emotional eating
- Chronic headaches
- Depression
- Diagnosis of anxiety or clinical depression
- Inability to concentrate
- Irritability
- Loss of interest in things you used to enjoy
- Mood swings
- Panic attacks
- Racing thoughts
- Sadness with no apparent cause

Beyond mood dysregulation, a hormone imbalance can also express physically. Are you experiencing any of the following?

- Changes in bleeding
- Hot flashes
- Low libido
- Night sweats, waking up drenched
- Tender breasts
- Water retention
- Weight gain in hips

Perimenopause typically begins in women in their 40s, but can start as early as the 30s or as late as the 50s. When it starts, it can really throw women for a loop. There's a sense of lack of control. Things are happening to your body unpredictably. And all this after spending your middle years settling into the rhythm of a monthly period. Even if you are told *"in your 40s, you'll experience night sweats,"* nothing can quite prepare you for waking up drenched. Let's examine the possible hormones that could be at the root of your mood dysregulation.

## STEROIDAL SEX HORMONES

Although there may be many reasons for mood changes that can be difficult to tease out, let's focus on the reproductive hormones, as they are a common and dramatic cause of mood swings and other mood issues, such as anxiety, depression, and irritability. Your levels of estrogen and progesterone can produce wildly different moods and symptoms, particularly depending on whether there is an excess or deficiency in either. Let's look at how this works.

### *ESTROGEN*

The hormone estrogen is responsible for female characteristics (breasts, fertility) along with a number of other actions including boosting blood flow to the brain and supporting nerve function. It is also intimately connected to serotonin, a neurotransmitter responsible for our moods of peace and happiness. When estrogen drops, so does serotonin, and thus our mood.

Physiologically, estrogen is produced primarily in the ovaries. However, as we age (approximately 35 and onward), the ovaries slow their production of estrogen, and in menopause the production ceases altogether. Estrogen's primary production organ then becomes the adrenal glands. (The same is true for progesterone.) Estrogen is also produced by adipose (fat) tissue, as well as in other ways. One way is through a conversion process of testosterone to estrogen (aromatization). This typically occurs when you are inflamed or insulin resistant. Estrogen can enter your body from the outside, either through eating phytoestrogens like soy or through exposure to xenoestrogens, which are synthetic or chemical compounds with estrogenic effects. These are present in many common items like skin care products, plastics (BPA), insecticides, and food additives (such as the preservative BHA and food dyes).

Another way that estrogen becomes dominant is when progesterone declines, so that while estrogen may not technically increase, it is in greater proportion to progesterone. This typically occurs when progesterone drops as you age. Progesterone declines at a faster rate than estrogen does, between the ages of 35 and 50. This results in a condition known as estrogen dominance. The symptoms can include mood swings, nervousness, anxiety, and irritability, as well as bloating and tender breasts, fibrocystic breasts, uterine fibroids, changes in your menstrual cycle, and weight gain, especially around your midsection.

Other reasons why estrogen can tip the scales in relation to progesterone include estrogen supplementation, a low-fiber diet, poor elimination (this can be a gut issue or liver congestion), nutrient deficiencies, and heavy metal toxicity.

On the flipside, if your estrogen is below optimal levels, you may begin to experience signs of estrogen deficiency. These can include hot flashes, night sweats, vaginal dryness, foggy thinking, memory lapses, mood swings (ding-ding-ding!)—such as feeling overly emotional, tearful, sad, or depressed—fatigue, incontinence, and trouble sleeping. Whether you're high or low in estrogen, examine your diet and lifestyle habits. Are you eating enough fat? Over-dieting? Are you experiencing chronic stress? Connecting the dots between how you're feeling and what you're doing will shorten your road to a more balanced existence.

Hormonious A-ha! If you're facing particularly demanding times in your life, this means that not only are your adrenals and your entire HPA axis being overly burdened, but you may have a more difficult transition into menopause. To remain symptom-free during this period and to maintain an even mood, do what you can to support your HPA axis. Recall the fight or flight response from Chapter 2 in stressful situations. The reproductive system shuts down while the body's sympathetic nervous system engages to defend itself for survival. Recall too, that DHEA, the hormone that balances cortisol, is the precursor to estrogen and testosterone, and progesterone is the precursor to cortisol. It's a web of interrelated hormones that can be affected not only by the body's natural aging process but by heightened stress.

Functional lab testing is another tool that can provide insight into how much estrogen the body is producing and how the body is processing it. The issue isn't just the level of hormones that you may have at any given time. It's also a matter of whether the body is processing the estrogen in ways that are helpful or harmful.

Unfortunately, we can't really prevent getting older, but we certainly can impact and control many factors that help right the tipping ship. Check out my Hormonious Tips along with my Fix Its at the end of this chapter.

### *PROGESTERONE*

Progesterone's main function is to balance estrogen. It also protects the nervous system by keeping levels of GABA (Gamma-aminobutyric acid, a neurotransmitter), circulating. GABA helps us feel relaxed and calm. When progesterone drops, so does GABA production, which may lead to feelings of irritability and anxiousness. This is another example of the intertwined relationship between the endocrine and neuroendocrine system. They are inextricably linked, therefore an impact in one will likely impact the other.

If deficient in progesterone, you may be having hot flashes, night sweats, or other sleep disturbances, vaginal dryness, foggy thinking, memory lapses, bone loss, incontinence, feeling tearful or depressed, and/or have heart palpitations.

If you have an excess, you may feel sleepy or be experiencing mild depression. You may also have a decreased libido, have breast swelling or tenderness, and may be susceptible to candida infections.

A balance between these hormones is important. If you have too much progesterone in relation to estrogen, you may be estrogen-deficient. Consult your physician to discuss ways to achieve optimum balance. I'll also address how these hormones can be managed in the Fix Its for this chapter.

### TESTOSTERONE

Both men and women have testosterone. This under-appreciated hormone boosts libido, builds bone, is important in cardiovascular health, and helps elevate mood. Even though women have less of it, it is still an important hormone in our systems and one that we neither want a deficiency or an excess of—it should be in balance with the other hormones because they all work together and are mutually influential. For example, excess facial hair isn't so much a result of excess testosterone as it is a reflection of deficient estrogen.

> **Hormonious Tip:** Cholesterol plays a critically important role in the production of sex hormones. It is the precursor to the hormone pregnenolone, which is the parent hormone to DHEA and progesterone. Recall that DHEA converts to estrogen and testosterone, and progesterone is the precursor to cortisol. This means that we want sufficient cholesterol to be able to convert to pregnenolone. Pregnenolone has been shown to improve mood, memory, and thinking, decrease symptoms of PMS, and aid in immune activity. Bottom line? Healthy fats are your friend. Those fat-free days are over and gone (thank goodness!).

> **Hormonious A-ha!** Do you experience hot flashes? This annoying and unpredictable heating up of the body is not only caused by imbalances of estrogen or progesterone. Caffeine can trigger hot flashes by increasing stress hormones. Remove coffee

and other caffeine sources for a time to see if your hot flash symptoms reduce. Thyroid disorders can also cause hot flashes.

## OTHER MOOD CULPRITS

### *THE DIGESTIVE TRACT AND YOUR MOOD*

The gut-brain connection is well documented, which is why the enteric nervous system (located along the length of the lining of the gastrointestinal system) is so often referred to as our second brain.[86] This "brain" has over 100 billion neurons (nervous system cells), and the gut contains almost every chemical substance that helps to run and control the brain, including neurotransmitters such as serotonin, dopamine, and norepinephrine. Did you know that 90% of serotonin in the body is produced in the gut? The gut also produces benzodiazepine, a chemical compound used as a psychoactive drug that enhances the effect of the neurotransmitter GABA. As a drug, it's a sedative used to combat anxiety, insomnia, seizures, and muscle spasms, but your healthy gut makes this chemical compound on its own! Considering the health of your digestive tract in juxtaposition to your moods, you can see why gut health is so crucial to healthy moods.

The health of your microbiome also influences your mood and "talks" to both the enteric nervous system and the brain. Beneficial bacteria support digestion, synthesize vitamins, produce serotonin, and help balance mood in many ways, like reducing anxiety. Any underlying dysbiosis (microbiome imbalance) can be the culprit when mood issues surface. Metabolites, or byproducts, of fungi and bacteria have been found in the urine of patients with various neurological conditions, including depression.[87] The following gut microbes in particular have been associated with dysbiosis:

- *Bacteroides fragilis*

- *Campylobacter jejuni*

- *Candida albicans* (commonly called "candida" or "yeast")

- *Candida tropicalis*

- *Citrobacter freundii*

- *Clostridium difficile*

- *Enterotoxigenic Escherichia coli*

- *Geotrichum spp.*

- *Klebsiella pneumoniae*

- *Proteus vulgaris*

Recall that some of the symptoms of a Candida or yeast overgrowth are related to mood disorders such as depression, anxiety, and irritability. Brain fog, an inability to concentrate, headaches, and migraines are also common symptoms of a Candida overgrowth.

## GOOD MOOD STARTS WITH GOOD FOOD

Hormones fluctuate and mess with your moods, but so does your dinner. What you eat not only impacts every cell in your body, but it can have a direct impact on your moods.[88] Recall the previous discussion on the importance of a level blood sugar to maintain steady energy? A blood sugar crash has the added side effect of mood dysregulation. That cupcake may taste delicious at the moment you're eating it, but when your mood dips shortly thereafter, that sugary, creamy, gluten-y treat played a starring role in taking you there and may be wreaking havoc elsewhere in your digestive system. As part of your efforts to stabilize your mood, you should avoid foods containing sugar and refined or heavily processed ingredients (white flour, for example) that cause blood sugar crashes. See the Fix Its section in this chapter for foods that promote a calm state of mind.

Unfortunately, there are foods that may be "good" but not for you. They may be causing a mood result—for example, mood swings, depression, anxiety, lightheadedness, headaches, feeling of fainting, or any number of varied emotional or physical symptoms and conditions. These are called trigger foods, and the process to determine whether they are a trigger for you is just that: a process.

Food sensitivity testing is available, but laboratories vary and results are not always conclusive. Nevertheless, it's a good option for efficiency purposes and provides a level of information that may be helpful for you.

More accurate is the process for evaluating whether these foods are a trigger for you, but this requires patience and daily journaling to keep track of reactions. The best way to do this is to eliminate trigger foods for about a month, then reintroduce them one at a time, carefully tracking any symptom recurrence. The most common trigger foods are the following, but this list is not exhaustive (it's possible that there is another food that doesn't agree with your system):

- Corn
- Dairy
- Eggs
- Fermented and old foods (like leftovers, especially meat), because of their histamine content
- Fish
- Milk (and other dairy products)
- Nightshade vegetables can cause an adverse reaction in some, and those with autoimmune conditions may be more susceptible. Common ones include: ashwagandha, bell peppers, cape gooseberries, eggplant, garden huckleberries, goji berries, hot peppers (e.g., chili, jalapeno, habanero, and scotch bonnet, as well as chili-based spices like cayenne, chili powder, crushed red pepper, and paprika), naranjillas, pepinos, pimentos, potatoes (except sweet potatoes), tomatillos, and tomatoes
- Peanuts
- Red meats

- Shellfish

- Soy

- Tree nuts

- Wheat

- Yeast

### SUGAR

Sugar. It's a sore subject because we have such a love affair with the stuff and tend to pursue it particularly for its opiate effect and its ability to temporarily improve poor mood. While sugar may provide a fleeting feeling of satisfaction, it's most often over-consumed, and consumed in a highly refined form, such as white sugar in cookies, muffins, and cakes, etc. Overeating these foods can result in a blood sugar spike and subsequent crash, thereby exacerbating any negative mood states. I personally pursued my path (in part) because I wanted to find healthy alternatives to sugar, especially since I inherited my mom's love for baking. But there's no way to put this gently: Refined sugar is damaging to your cells, addictive, and an anti-nutrient. That is, it requires more nutrients for the body to process it than what it supplies. Sugar is literally the opposite of what your body needs to be healthy, and the more you eat, the more your brain is triggered to want more. It accelerates aging, increases wrinkling and sagging of skin, and causes bloating, fat retention, and an imbalanced microbiome. Too much sugar, especially white table sugar, can interfere with leptin, the hormone that regulates appetite (more on leptin in Chapter 6).

Take note of my steps in the following section to reduce your intake of sugar. If sugar continues to be a problem for you, and your cravings are ruling your snack or meal choices, investigate whether Candida overgrowth is an issue for you. For further discussion on cravings, see Chapter 2.

**Hormonious Tip:** The B-complex vitamins have dramatic mood-elevating effects—more so than almost any other nutrient. B vitamins are critical for the efficient liver detoxification of unwanted chemicals such as heavy metals, histamines, and bacterial toxins that could be at the root of your immune or neurological challenges. The complex of B vitamins is crucial for nerve function and nerve cell metabolism, which produce optimal neurotransmitter levels.

**Hormonious Tip:** Low levels of these vitamins and minerals can impact your hormones and mood. Corresponding food suggestions can be found in this chapter's Fix Its.

- **Vitamin B12 (Cobalamin)** is an essential element responsible for mood balance, playing a vital role in nervous system function. Low levels can cause fatigue, impaired reasoning, and depression.

- **Vitamin C** supports mood balance, brain health, and nervous system health. This essential vitamin reduces stress and anxiety and serves to provide antioxidant protection.[89] (Antioxidants are discussed in Chapter 6.)

- **Calcium.** If you're experiencing PMS-related depression, you may be calcium deficient. In addition to its role in maintaining strong bones and teeth, calcium is responsible for preserving healthy muscle and nerve function and supporting the absorption process of Vitamin B12.

- **Chromium** is a trace mineral and you only need small amounts. Without it, however, your body will have difficulty regulating insulin. Chromium aids in the production of serotonin, norepinephrine, and melatonin, which are each involved in helping the brain regulate mood and emotion.

- **Folate (Vitamin B9 or folic acid)** supports reproductive health and regulates serotonin. This supplement is sometimes paired with Vitamin B12 to treat depression.

- **Iron.** If you are deficient in iron, you may experience fatigue or depression. Iron supports energy and transports oxygen.

- **Magnesium** is one of the most important minerals our body needs for good mood. A deficiency can cause irritability, fatigue, and stress.

# FIX IT

The answers to tackling your moods are many and multi-dimensional. Chances are, multiple causes have contributed, including external stressors, internal stressors and bad habits as well as that notorious culprit, hormone imbalance. While the body's complicated circuitry may be readjusting and your mood is being impacted, your ability to weather the storm by reframing negative thought patterns and replacing bad health habits with good ones will certainly be beneficial. Review your FTP and notice whether there is a corresponding event, trigger, or any other factor possibly at play in your life right now. This is an opportunity to look upstream at possible culprits and determine whether a particular recommendation resonates with you.

## What to Do

### *Power your mood (to good) through movement.*
Exercise is essential to maintaining hormone balance and keeping depression and anxiety at bay. It also helps regulate estrogen and progesterone levels in premenopausal women.[90] Moving your body is simply a powerful way to feel good. It boosts your brain's dopamine, norepinephrine, and serotonin levels, all of which impact your mood for the better. Not to mention releasing those feel-good endorphins!

For those who are accustomed to a sedentary lifestyle, start with walking. Open your door, step outside, and stretch your arms up towards the sky. Dress warm for inclement weather and begin your walk around the block. It's refreshing, free, and easy, and you can do it anytime. Make this a daily habit and build up the length of your walks over several weeks. Start by walking only a few minutes a day—that's it to start. Make sure to walk with intention and energy, and feel the earth (sidewalk) under your feet. Once you develop the habit of walking outdoors, increase the amount of time you spend. Raise the time level each week. Aim for 30 minutes and progress to longer. The name of the game is movement. Even if you don't feel like it, this one constant can provide a lifeline while you're untangling the rest of yourself from its moody place. No prescription needed.

For those who are already engaged in a routine, change it up and try something new:

- Aerial silk, which is a form of flexibility acrobat training using long silk fabric for support and stretching. It's as fun as it sounds!

- Barre class

- Boxing

- Dancing (take a tango, hip-hop, or ballet class)

- HIIT (high intensity interval training) supports weight loss far better than endurance cardio. These are short bursts of training, where you exercise at high intensity for 30 to 60 seconds followed by a period of 30 to 60 seconds of rest.[91]

- Kickboxing

- Pickle ball

- Pilates

- Spinning

- Swimming

- Tai chi

- TRX (total resistance exercise, which is a form of suspension training)

- Yoga or hot yoga

A localized Google search will uncover new possibilities in your neighborhood. In addition to working out locally, ClassPass, Flywheel, and DailyBurn offer you the opportunity to exercise in your own home with live streaming workouts. The trend in exercise is always finding new ways to move your body that are fun and invigorating. Mix it up and rotate your workouts to keep yourself interested. Alternate which muscles you are working for the best overall fitness and reduced chance of injury. Your mood and your brain will both thank you.

Options to incorporate exercise into your workday are plentiful. Most major cities offer bike lanes for those who want to ride to work. Downtown office buildings and suburban corporate offices contain gyms or clubs. And if you don't have access to an exercise gym during your workday, there are plenty of ways to get movement at your desk. The under-desk elliptical device engages you to perform elliptical movements while sitting at your desk. Other devices force your body to experience micromovements, which energize and wake up passive muscles, such as the motion board for standing or the motion stool for sitting. The motion stool provides stability plus active sitting, working muscles you rarely engage. Keeping a few hand weights in your work area means that you can work on muscle building as well.

Movement doesn't have to only take the form of organized exercise. Walking, hiking, cross-country skiing, bike riding, even taking your dog for a run or playing a friendly game of soccer with your kids at the park are ways to activate your senses and release the feel-good endorphins that make exercise essential for elevating mood.

Hormonious Tip: Keep track of your movement with your smartphone or other wearable device. Here are a few options, which include app integrations to explore (these devices were available at the writing of this book):

- Apple Watch
- Bellabeat Wellness Coach
- FitBit
- Garmin Connect
- Workout for Women
- Back Neck & Posture: MoovBuddy

Don't want to wear a device? Check out the app Sweatcoin that pays you for walking. How's that for incentive?

### *Evaluate your sleep.*

Getting good sleep is critical to a balanced mood. If you're not getting enough of it, this very well could be contributing to your mood dysregulation. Human growth hormone (HGH; discussed further in Chapter 6) is produced when you sleep, and if you're deficient in HGH, your mood will be impacted too. If sleep is at all an issue for you, make sure to reread Chapter 3 and the corresponding Fix Its section.

### *Participate in activities that make you happy.*

Make a list of all the things that you have always enjoyed doing. Select something from that list and engage in that activity. If nothing on that list is speaking to you right now, then get creative and think about what would fill you up. When I was depressed, I purchased paint and small canvases and experimented with painting both in my home and at the nearby botanical gardens. It was something I always wanted to do but had never done before. It was therapeutic and filled me with uber satisfaction. It reminded me that there are ways to engage in the world that are uplifting even if our mood tells us otherwise. When the right thing comes to you, you'll experience a zing or vibration in your body telling you, "This is the thing! This is what I want to try/do." Here are a few ideas for you to consider:

- Listen to music, sing a song
- Paint, sculpt, draw
- Knit, needlepoint, collage
- Use the app Lake to create colorful works of art
- Learn how to play a new game like mahjong, euchre, poker, bridge, canasta
- Create a new recipe
- Write a poem
- Listen to comedy
- Research a place you want to visit or travel to
- Learn a new language
- Invent a product that fixes a problem
- Learn how to invest
- Take up photography
- Learn a new sport
- Pot a plant or take up gardening
- Take an acting class
- Spend time in a craft store, home building store, or other retail environment that gives you a bounce in your step. The local hardware store could be the perfect place to start.
- Still not sure? Get quiet to find your next spirit-lifting pursuit.

### *Examine your closest relationships.*

Are you involved in a relationship that is respectful, mutual, and balanced? Does it fill you up? If you are dissatisfied with some aspect, spend some time journaling to get clear on what the challenges are. Consider discussing these things with your partner to find common ground. Recognize that if your mood is imbalanced, this is a topic worth introducing into your conversations. Understanding where you're at in this moment can help your partner set expectations.

### *Spend time with friends to brighten your mood.*

Starved for connection? Your social connections are foundational to good health and can be more restorative to your healing process than one ideal meal. Reconnect with an old friend or make new ones by joining an organization that you want to affiliate with, one that will enrich your soul and deepen your connection to your purpose. Spending time with good friends who live far away can be arranged by either a phone call, Skype session, or planning for a much-needed girl get-away. Your girlfriends (and guy friends) are your support heroes, and spending time with them will help shake you out of and distract you from your bad mood. One great way to spend time with friends is through game play, mentioned previously. This not only works your brain, but the social aspect can lift your mood.

### *Compare yourself to yourself.*

This culture is abundantly engaged with technology, and often to your detriment. It not only interferes with precious time that could be spent bettering yourself but can serve as a negative distraction. Be aware of your thoughts as you engage in social media. Where does technology and social media fit into your life? And more specifically, is it interfering with your sense of self? Observing the life of others is fine provided that you don't compare yourself to anyone other than yourself. Instead, compare yourself to yourself, at different points in time or if mastering a new skill. Adopt this concept and use it globally in your interactions or outside of them, so that your thoughts are founded without judgment towards yourself. Rather, reflect on what it is you would like to change, if anything, and go about making those changes.

***Volunteer to overcome mood and stress and #BeAJoyfulWarrior*[92]**

During periods of chronic stress or fatigue, you may see a decrease in mood, as well as a decrease in estrogen, progesterone, and testosterone. (Yet again, here is an example of the interconnectedness of your body's processes.) Engage in activities that will lift your mood and relieve stress for better mood and hormonal balance. One of the best ways to shake mood is to help someone else improve their situation or feel better. This is akin to feeling grateful for what you have and where you're at in life.

It also provides you an opportunity to give your time and share yourself, elevating positive feelings and lifting your sweet spirit. Consider serving in one of these areas:

- Animal rescue shelters
- Children and teen support groups
- Environmental organizations
- Hospitals or hospices
- Retirement or nursing homes
- Veterans organizations
- Women's shelters

If none of the above resonate with you, research one that does. There are plenty of people or organizations who would love your help, and who will help you feel better when you give your time to them. If volunteer work does not align with your interests, consider other ways to engage with your community, your neighbors, or your home. For example, maybe an elderly neighbor has few visitors and would love your company. Or perhaps your area has a women's group you can join.

***Connect with your roots.***

Nothing satisfies quite like learning more about and connecting with your past. You are a link in a long chain, and learning about where you came from and how you came to be is a fascinating story. As you dig, you may learn about relatives who have similar traits. These could provide insights into how you want to live your life today. This exploration into the generations that came before is a strategy to ground you in the present, and to give your life meaning. If you are adopted and interested in learning about your biological parents, or not, you are here for a reason, and you've got a story to share. Determine whether learning about your biological roots fits into your current life goals.

And on that note, I encourage you to write your story. Maybe you're thinking "I don't have a story," or "My life isn't that interesting." Guess what? It is, because it belongs to you, and you get to write the ending to it. You get to decide what happens next, who you want to be, and where you want to go. This is no light-hearted directive. I realize this may stir in you uncomfortable feelings. That is partly the point. Discomfort is a starting point for something better, and writing this out is part of your pilgrimage to health. Your health journey is tied to your life journey. In some ways, the two are tangled together. Your health is your life right now, and your life is your health. Do you see the connection?

If your efforts become halted or delayed, that's okay. But I respectfully invite you to come back to this offer. This is no simple request to exercise more. This is a way to build deeper meaning into your life, and one way to do this is to get to know yourself better by exploring the roots of your family's origins, culture, language, and rich history. This process may inspire you to consider family recipes that have been passed down through generations. Spend time by creating a healthier version, which is a sure way to boost your mood.

***Be kind to yourself.***

**"This is where I'm at"** was my trademark mantra when I was walking my way through stress, anxiety, and depression. Focus on a point in front of you—something that you would like to do, learn, explore, or change—and hold this thought as the light at the end of your proverbial tunnel. Wherever you are in your struggle to feel better, be kind and gentle with yourself. Accept this moment without shame, and let the idea wash over you that you will be stronger when you are on the other side of this, but for now, your body is in need of nurture and support. While your mind may try, don't engage in negative self-talk. Rather, impose the rule that wherever you are is a non-judgment zone. To that end, as well as you possibly can, surround yourself with those who love and support you.

The concept of *"This is where I'm at"* can be used as a meditation tool as well. Think of a place where you have spent time feeling positive and joyful, or that evokes feelings of calm, light, and soothing comfort. It could be a place that you have traveled to, a memory from an earlier time, or a favorite setting in your imagination, like a forested mountain range, rippling ocean waves, or a multi-colored sky above a setting sun. Use this image when you find yourself in a gloomy mood. Close your eyes and imagine yourself in this place. Breathe in the smells. Add into this picture any elements that will bring it alive in your mind. Are there people there? Or, are you alone? Are you standing? Sitting? Do birds fly by? Is the mountain covered in snow, the ocean calm, the sunset orange? What can you hear, smell, feel? Activate all your senses in service of this visualization. Spending time in this space can help you reframe your mood by reframing your thoughts.

Finally, remember that this is a process and may take practice, but keep at it. It's an enjoyable and incredibly beneficial exercise.

### Care for your digestive tract.
When your mood is out of balance, remember the importance of the health of your digestive tract for your mood and the gut-brain connection—the gut and brain are inextricably linked. That means

inflammation in the gut—for example leaky gut or dysbiosis—can cause inflammation in the brain.[93] When unfriendly bacteria exceed the good bacteria they produce neurotoxins, which not only can slow your ability to think or retain information, but can also trigger depression. Since most of your serotonin (your feel-good hormone) is produced in your gut, you want to make sure you're treating it well. Assess the foods that you eat regularly. Are they inflammatory? Is it possible you are eating a food to which you're sensitive? Nourishing your GI can directly improve your mood. Get that serotonin back in circulation!

Also, consider that you should be pooping once a day at minimum, especially if your moods are irregular. Not doing so indicates a backup in the system and that toxins (including excess estrogen) that should be removed daily could be reabsorbing and recirculating. You want your bowels to clear excess estrogen. Support them and your colon by making sure that you are eating sufficient sources of fiber. Supplement as needed to establish regularity.

### Embrace solitude.

I am a big believer that time alone can be incredibly powerful for your mood. The reverse can also be true. If you are in a place of sadness and low spirits, spending time with others may be more appropriate until you right your ship. But when you are feeling that your mood has crossed the line to the neutral or positive side of the scale, time alone can help grow your mood even more. While many women find the idea of solo travel scary and unappealing, it actually can be quite empowering, uplifting, and even life changing. But you don't have to set out globetrotting to get a taste of alone time. Solitude can be a simple walk through a park, but it can also be a weekend away. It can be exploring a new or nearby city, journaling in a local coffee shop, challenging the cultural standard by dining alone or watching a movie by yourself! These can all inspire a fresh perspective from which to examine your role in life, and the story that has gotten you here. Perhaps it's time for a new chapter? A new beginning? A new way of interacting with the world and those around you?

There are many ways to cross that bridge of discomfort and overcome the voice of fear that is interfering with what's possible. The *you* that's in there is looking for another way to express herself, relieve that burdensome mood slump, and kick it into another gear. One way to overcome that old, nervy fear is to ponder the following question: What is the worst that can happen? However you answer this, remember my initial prompt to you: What is your 90 year old self telling you to do?

### *Engage support.*

1.  Visit your doctor to initiate a discussion about your mood. If you were my client, I would be asking you detailed questions such as:
    a.  What kind of mood state are you in?
    b.  When did this start?
    c.  How long has this been going on?
    d.  Was there a triggering event?
    e.  What have you been doing that has worked? Hasn't worked?

2.  Talk with your spouse, partner, loved ones, and friends. Tell them what you are dealing with right now and ask for their understanding and guidance.

3.  The Profile of Mood States is a questionnaire that provides a rating scale of mood states. Use it as a reference guide to help articulate your particular moods—you can find the link in the Resources section. If you are experiencing depression or anxiety, there are several organizations that you can reach out to. Some can provide free evaluations.
    a.  National Alliance on Mental Illness (NAMI):

https://www.nami.org/

b. Anxiety and Depression Association of America: https://adaa.org

c. American Foundation for Suicide Prevention: https://afsp.org/

d. Freedom From Fear: http://www.freedomfromfear. org

**Hormonious A-ha! And a Purposeful Life.** Through the process of untangling the source of your mood imbalance, please give thought to your purpose here on earth. What is it? What are you meant to do while you're here? What impact can you make or do you want to make? In this case, size doesn't matter. Your 'Why' can be whatever you want it to be because this is your life and you get to decide how you want to be in it. Maybe you're already living your purpose. But underneath this question is a river of possibility and ideas that will welcome your consideration, particularly if this idea is at all related to your mood imbalance. There are ways that you can become an integral part of something essential. This can support your efforts to feel more meaning and purpose in your life. Review the previously mentioned Fix Its for ideas. Where your attention goes, your mood will follow. Focus your attention on something that satisfies your soul. Want a little guidance into how your unique personality profile can support your efforts? Check out https://www.16personalities.com to do just that.

# WHAT TO EAT

### *Balance your blood sugar.*
Ensure that your meals are a nice balance of fat, fiber (a type of carbohydrate), and protein, to avoid the highs and lows that throw off your blood sugar balance and contribute to feelings of irritability, tiredness, and other off-putting negative moods.

### *Eat healthy fats to build your hormones.*

- Avocados
- Butter/ghee (if you are not sensitive to dairy, and only from organic sources; ghee is butter with the solids removed and may be okay for those who are lactose intolerant)
- Coconut or MCT oils
- Fish oil (from supplements as well as fatty fish like salmon)
- Meat from grass-fed/pasture-raised animals
- Nuts like walnuts and almonds
- Olive oil (extra virgin = unrefined and cold pressed, so the oil retains its nutritional benefits)
- Seeds like chia and flaxseeds

### *Add good-mood-promoting nutrients.*

- Eat nourishing fermented foods that will enrich your microbiome and help ease negative moods. See Chapter 2 and the Resources for more information.
- Vitamins B6, B9, and B12 support mood balance.
- Omega-3-rich foods (like fatty fish and flaxseed)
- Vitamin B6 (Pyridoxine) foods:
    - Bananas
    - Beef
    - Chicken
    - Potatoes
    - Salmon
    - Spinach

- o   Sunflower seeds
- o   Sweet potatoes
- o   Tuna
- o   Turkey
- Vitamin B9 (Folate) foods
  - o   Asparagus
  - o   Beans (black, garbanzo, kidney, navy, pinto, etc.)
  - o   Broccoli
  - o   Dark leafy greens (spinach, turnip greens, etc.)
  - o   Lentils
- Vitamin B12 (Cobalamin) foods

The highest[94] Cobalamin contents are contained in the following foods in micrograms (mcg) per 3 ½ ounces:

- o   Lamb liver 104.0
- o   Clams 98.0
- o   Beef liver 80.0
- o   Lamb kidneys 63.0
- o   Calf liver 60.0
- o   Beef kidneys 31.0
- o   Chicken liver 25.0
- o   Oysters 18.0
- o   Sardines 17.0
- o   Beef heart 11.0
- o   Egg yolks 6.0
- o   Lamb heart 5.2
- o   Trout 5.0

Plus, the following:

- o   Brains, all kinds (4.0)

- o   Cheese
- o   Chicken
- o   Cod
- o   Crab
- o   Eggs
- o   Mackerel
- o   Milk (cow)
- o   Mussels
- o   Rockfish
- o   Salmon
- o   Scallops
- o   Shrimp
- o   Tuna
- o   Turkey
- o   Yogurt
- Vitamin C foods
  - o   Bell peppers
  - o   Broccoli
  - o   Brussels sprouts
  - o   Cabbage
  - o   Cantaloupe
  - o   Cauliflower
  - o   Dark leafy greens
  - o   Grapefruit
  - o   Kiwi
  - o   Lemons
  - o   Limes
  - o   Oranges

- o Papaya
- o Pineapple
- o Potatoes
- o Spinach
- o Strawberries
- o Sweet red peppers
- o Tomatoes
- Calcium-rich foods
  - o Dark leafy greens (collard greens, kale, mustard greens, spinach, turnip greens, etc.)
  - o Organically sourced tofu
  - o Organic or raw cheese that is free of hormones
  - o Sardines
  - o Sesame seeds
  - o Yogurt
- Chromium foods
  - o Black pepper
  - o Broccoli
  - o Green beans
  - o Romaine lettuce
  - o Oats
  - o Tomatoes
- Iron foods
  - o Asparagus
  - o Beans
  - o Bok choy
  - o Cumin
  - o Dark leafy greens (collard greens, spinach, Swiss

chard, etc.)

- o Eggs
- o Leeks
- o Lentils
- o Organ meats
- o Parsley
- o Poultry
- o Red meats
- o Shellfish
- o Turmeric
- Magnesium foods
    - o Beans (black, navy, soy)
    - o Cashews
    - o Dark leafy greens (spinach, kale, Swiss chard, etc.)
    - o Quinoa
    - o Seeds (pumpkin, sesame, sunflower)

### Drink Lion's Mane mushroom tea.

Japanese researchers found that Lion's Mane mushroom reduces depression and anxiety in a period of four weeks.[95] Though originally used primarily for digestive health, this mushroom is now well known for its important brain health properties, specifically its ability to protect the myelin sheath that surrounds nerve fibers[96] (the breakdown of which occurs in Alzheimer's). Its benefits to the brain are fascinating and worth a cup or two. You can even grow Lion's Mane mushrooms at home.

### Review the Fix Its in the other chapters.

Many of the Fix Its in other sections of this book will support you through your mood issues. Start your review with Chapter 2.

# WHAT TO AVOID

### *Alcohol*

Alcohol, such as red wine (which contains brain-friendly antioxidants and resveratrol, a phytonutrient that helps to relax the blood vessels), still contains sugar. Sugar and an imbalanced mood are not a good pair. Alcohol is also inflammatory to the intestines, hard on the liver, and most importantly, not a good friend to you when your mood is uneven (even if you think it's all you need to cheer up!). Though the liver breaks down most of the alcohol a person consumes, the process of that breakdown creates toxins that are inflammatory and weaken the immune system. If you are drinking alcohol to calm your mood, there are other alternatives; see the recommended supplements in the following "What to Take" section. Alcohol also suppresses melatonin, the sleep hormone.

I realize the implications in my making this recommendation. You are likely rolling your eyes, or thinking, "Yeah, right, Karen, like I'm going to give up my wine!" I understand. Completely. I'm not asking you to give up alcohol forever. I'm asking you to take a break, a vacation of sorts, so that you can see how alcohol may be worsening your moods and disrupting your hormone balance. Aim for 30 days. If that seems too long, find a length of time that you are willing to try living without alcohol. Start with a week, or even a weekend. The social aspects of alcohol are pervasive in our culture and society, and going out with friends means that you might get eyeballed or questioned. If this is too challenging for you, evaluate how much alcohol you drink per week and see if you can institute guidelines for yourself to moderate your intake, such as allowing yourself one glass of red or white wine once on the weekend, but never during the week.

You could also consider upgrading the wine that you drink by choosing organic wines. You'll be doing your body good in several ways, including reducing the pesticide residue that's attached to the grapes as well as the additives that many U.S. wine growers use to make their wine. Additives can be defoaming agents, artificial coloring, extra sugar, high-fructose corn syrup, ammonia, and genetically modified bacteria and yeasts. Since wine producers are not required to disclose any of these on the bottle, you could very well be drinking a wine that is really doing your body harm. Companies like Dry Farm Wines are committed to representing organic growers, along with their philosophy that good wine need not be overly high in alcohol content, thereby eliminating tomorrow's hangover. See the Resources for a link to get a bottle of their wine for a penny.

### Caffeine

If you are a coffee drinker and experience any of the symptoms mentioned at the outset of this chapter, consider removing caffeine for a time until your symptoms resolve and you determine the root cause of your health imbalance. Caffeine is a stimulant and can exacerbate feelings of anxiousness, nervousness, and irritability. The ups and downs can also contribute to dehydration, blood sugar swings, and cravings. Caffeine can deplete the body of nutrients, particularly when taken with meals.

But quitting cold turkey is no picnic, and believe it or not, that is not the best method.

It's best to taper off in small increments so as not to trigger the junkie-like symptoms many people struggle with. Slowly dialing down the caffeine allows your body to acclimate.

Here's a painless strategy[97] to try when you're ready to unhook from the caffeine drip:

- Day 1: Today, have your usual amount of coffee.

- Day 2 to Day 5: Blend your coffee 50/50 with decaf (preferably certified organic).

- Day 6: Blend your coffee 25/75 with decaf (see note above).

- Day 7: Start drinking pure decaf or switch to green tea.

# WHAT TO TAKE

### *Probiotics will support your gut garden and can reduce anxiety and stress.*

(See page 84 for more information.) Consider probiotics that include the species *Lactobacillus rhamnosus*. This probiotic bacterium contains the neurotransmitter GABA, helping to regulate brain activity and calm anxiety.[98]

### *All Vitamin Bs play an important role in mood balance.*

A deficiency in any of them can be a cause of depression. A standard CBC blood test from your doctor can reveal whether you might be low on some of these vitamins. If you are eating sufficient amounts of food containing Vitamin B12 or you are supplementing, yet still have low levels, consider low stomach acid as a possible underlying cause. Another factor could be absorption issues, for which there are many possible explanations. For example, mercury (from too much fish or other sources) can inhibit the absorption of Vitamin B12, among other nutrients. Review Chapter 2 for ways to shore this up.

### *Love your liver.*

Consider incorporating a supplement that supports healthy liver function. When your liver is taxed and overburdened, your entire system slows down, and toxins (including excess estrogen) get recirculated. *Yuck.* Look for herbal blends that contain milk thistle, dandelion root, and other herbs like turmeric, barberry (root bark), or ginger. Keep an eye out for N-Acetyl Cysteine (NAC) and L-Methionine in a liver support supplement. These are amino acids known to enhance the liver's production of glutathione. Glutathione is essential to the liver's detoxification process.

### *Magnesium (See page 152 for direction.)*

Consider using magnesium citrate if you are constipated as it has a laxative effect.

### *5-HTP*

5-HTP (5-Hydroxytryptophan) is an amino acid and a precursor to serotonin. It is often recommended in cases of sleep disorders, depression, and anxiety. Due to the possible accompanying side effects, 5-HTP should only be considered in consultation with your doctor.

### *Triphala*

An Ayurvedic herbal remedy that helps with constipation,[99] triphala is made from three different berries. It's anti-inflammatory, has anti-oxidative properties, and may aid in weight loss.[100]

> Hormonious Tip: Pay attention to CBD (cannabidiol) oil. It is gaining acceptance and being used to treat a wide assortment of ailments, including anxiety[101] and sleep disorders.[102] CBD is a derivative of the cannabis plant (marijuana), which is rich in chemicals called cannabinoids. These cannabinoids attach to special receptors in the brain. You're probably familiar with THC (tetrahydrocannabinol), the cannabinoid responsible for the "high" effect. CBD is another cannabinoid but doesn't produce a high. Due to its popularity, CBD continues to be studied and researched.

My Favorite[!] recipe is on the next page!

## RECIPE: SIMPLIFY TRUFFLES

Sometimes, a girl just needs a little chocolate to cheer her up. Here's where I turn when my sweet tooth threatens to disrupt my good intentions.

### Ingredients

1/2 cup almond butter

1/2 cup cashew butter

1/2 cup raw cacao nibs, divided

1/4 cup dried unsweetened cherries

4 dates pitted (soak in water to soften)

1 to 2 tablespoons ground flaxseed

1 teaspoon vanilla

1 teaspoon cinnamon

Dash of sea salt

### Method

In a food processor, blend almond butter, cashew butter, 1/4 cup of the cacao nibs, cherries, dates, flaxseed, vanilla, cinnamon, and salt. Set aside.

- Wearing rubber gloves, roll almond butter mixture into 1-inch balls. Roll the balls in cacao nibs.

- Keep frozen or in the fridge.

- Treat yourself to one with a hot cup of chamomile tea.

### Add-ins and Substitutions

- Use currants or other dried, unsweetened fruit.

- Truffles can alternatively be rolled in raw cacao powder or unsweetened coconut flakes.

- This recipe can be easily doubled, tripled, etc.

I named these beauties after a song called "Simplify" by Brendan James. Check it out here: http://bit.ly/2sbzHuv.

# CHAPTER 6

# HOW WEIGHT LOSS #RESISTS

*"The food choices we make matter down to the mitochondria."*
*—Andrea Nakayama*

There are many reasons why women gain weight, and many other reasons why they suddenly find themselves unable to lose it, but the underlying cause of your weight(y) conundrum may very well be related to hormone dysregulation. If you suffer from digestive issues, stress, poor sleep, and/or mood issues, you are likely to have struggles with your weight as well, and hormones are either the primary culprit or at least an aider and abettor.

The topic of food and what to eat is a complicated one. There is a lot of information out there, and on top of that, we all have attached our feelings, emotions, nostalgic (or traumatic) experiences, and habits to the supposedly simple act of eating. Now, as we reach a certain age, we also find that we cannot eat the way we did when we were children or young adults, meaning the ways we used to lose weight probably don't work so well anymore. Our food supply has also changed, and not necessarily for the better. So what are we to do if we know we need to lose weight, not even for vanity, but for health and longevity?

Renovating your eating habits is not easy but the payoff is large. Food is meant to nourish your cells and keep you healthy. The taste, flavors, and textures are also meant to satisfy your senses. But we use food in many other ways and put a lot of baggage onto our plates along with our dinners (and especially our desserts).

What I ask you to do to kick off this chapter is just one simple thing: At every meal, consider the food in front of you. Is it nutritious, or just "fun?" Think about that, and why you might choose something that does not nourish you in favor of something that hurts you. It's a simple question, really.

The truth is, none of us are going to "eat clean" 100% of the time. I certainly don't and I don't ask you to either. Eating clean means every food that you eat came from organic, pasture-raised, or wild-caught sources; it means not dipping into foods that are devoid of nutrients and raise and drop your blood sugar like bagels, bread, cookies, and so on. It means thinking about the origins of your food and how it came to be on your plate, such as whether pesticides or other chemicals played a part. It also means consciously choosing the highest quality food you possibly can for your circumstances. In other words, it is to a large degree a definition that you can create for yourself, as long as it is about quality, purity, and nutrition.

The most important thing I would like you to do is to think carefully about your expectations for the foods you choose to eat. What do you want food to do for you? What do you want this book to do for you? What do you want out of your health efforts? If it's something more than business as usual, then the simple reality is that you are probably going to need to make some changes, and those changes start with awareness. Awareness of what you choose to eat, awareness of what those choices mean for your health, and also, awareness of how our society attempts to get you to eat what is profitable rather than what is nutritious.

It's rare to avoid being bombarded with advertisements for fast food, sugary sodas, desserts, and all the other packaged, processed iterations of SAD (standard American diet) food. Dig a little deeper and you'll learn that our soil is being depleted, which means even our natural whole foods are less nutritious than they once were. There are more chemicals in the environment now than ever before, which means your body has to work harder to remove the toxins. Technology has entered our lives in a way that has made us sedentary, and many of us are still struggling to understand how to co-exist with that reality. Finally, stress has perhaps never been as pervasive in a non-war situation as it is today. It seems, ironically, that the easier life gets, the harder it is to cope.

This is a good time to take another look back at your Functional Timeline Plus, specifically with an eye for what in your past and present may be causing weight gain and/or inhibiting weight loss. Remember that there is a complexity at play here that may require some analysis. You may already know this, but "eating less and exercising more" is just one tiny part of the picture. Look at your story, and then follow the steps laid out for you in this chapter, and you can tackle your weight issues with more complete knowledge and an individualized perspective that generic diet plans simply can't offer. Whether you have suddenly added on extra pounds, have been trying to lose weight but it keeps sticking, or you can't stop eating, there is a path for you to understand what's going on and to take steps to getting to healthier.

Let's begin with a client of mine whose genetics served her for most of her life...until she hit perimenopause.

Caroline, who had just turned 53, came to me desperate to lose weight. In our first session, she showed me photographs of herself taken only a few years prior, when she was at a significantly lower weight. While Caroline's diet needed an update, I immediately saw that this was just a small part of her problem. In addition to her lack of exercise, Caroline's age meant that she was going through perimenopause and that her hormonal fluctuations were likely contributing significantly to her struggle. Remember the term "metabolic chaos?" When your hormones are driving the bus and you are in the backseat, a coup may be in order—but it will have to be a strategic one.

## HORMONAL WEIGHT ISSUE #1: DIET AND EXERCISE

Let's start with Caroline's diet. For her, a typical day consisted of cereal with fruit or a bagel with cream cheese for breakfast; a sandwich with chips for lunch; pasta or chicken and rice for dinner. Snacks and desserts were everyday occurrences, and red wine was a standard evening affair. She rarely ate fruit or vegetables other than the occasional side salad, and she didn't exercise. Although her nutrient-poor diet and lack of movement are classic symptoms of weight gain, these elements had not been an issue for Caroline in the past. Lucky Caroline for all those years! Yet, although her habits hadn't changed, her hormones had. There were several things I wanted to try with Caroline. The first was to educate her about how her food choices were impacting her, down to a cellular level. Later in this chapter, I'll share with you exactly what I showed her. The second was to help her make small changes in her diet that would cause big cellular changes, moving her towards both better health and easier weight loss. Then there was that business of not exercising. The free ride was over for Caroline (and may be over for you, if you are sedentary). Lack of exercise is not only a major cause of chronic disease[103] but certainly a contributing factor to weight loss resistance. Bottom line, especially in perimenopause (and any "-pause"): If you're not moving, your weight won't either.

## HORMONAL WEIGHT ISSUE #2: INFLAMMATION

Eating less and exercising more was (again) only part of the story for Caroline (and likely for you, too). Another very common issue at play in cases of weight loss resistance is inflammation. Caroline was eating many inflammatory foods and practicing inflammatory lifestyle behaviors, and I knew she would have to reduce these to see success. The first step was removing highly inflammatory foods. At first, Caroline was afraid she would be hungry all the time if she gave up the inflammatory Most Wanted list of foods: sugar, white flour, anything containing gluten, dairy products, and anything in a package with more than three ingredients. But once she started to make these changes and try new ways of eating, she not only felt good physically, she felt good about the way these changes were impacting her emotionally. And she was not hungry! Her mood brightened and she was joyful but most importantly, she felt that she understood how her choices were impacting her, and that when she occasionally dipped into her old way of eating, how that made her feel too. She appreciated the fact that I never told her "*do not eat those [bad] things again.*" Rather, I instructed her to be present and mindful of why she was eating something in particular, how it made her feel, and ultimately, to accept that it was okay to not eat perfectly, but that what really matters is what you do most of the time. Added bonus: She got much more creative in her meal-making and tried many new foods that she discovered she loved.

## HORMONAL WEIGHT ISSUE #3: HORMONAL CHANGES

I also did some testing on Caroline to determine her hormonal situation, but even without it, her irregular cycle was evidence that she was heading towards menopause. When estrogen rises (estrogen dominance) and then drops (estrogen deficiency) in those years prior to the final end of the menstrual cycle, many systems in the body are affected, including blood sugar/insulin balance, leptin and ghrelin levels, thyroid hormones, and more. Remember, every system in your body is interconnected, and when one thing changes, many other things change downstream and may have already changed upstream. This was key in my selection of the types of nutrient-dense foods I recommended for Caroline so she could actively provide her cells with the nutrients they needed for the healthiest possible hormonal transition.

Once Caroline got into the swing of making these additions and replacing the bad with much better options, she began to lose weight, finally, slowly but steadily (and not overnight). I'm not a patient person myself, so I get that this may be frustrating to hear, but the truth is that permanent weight loss takes time. It's a #step-bystep affair that requires building up the relationship that rules all else—the one you have with yourself.

Caroline's process for eliminating highly processed and refined foods and replacing them with nutrient-dense ones, along with implementing various lifestyle upgrades like more exercise and more active stress management, were ultimately the reasons for her success, not just because she was "eating less" and "exercising more" but because she was rebalancing her out-of-balance system, stabilizing her blood sugar, and feeding her cells with the nutrients necessary for health optimization. Her body was finally getting the nourishment it craved. She now understood how the choices she had made in the past were inflaming her body.

These newfound feelings supported Caroline's challenge with exercise. For someone who has never exercised, starting was a struggle. As you've read in this book, walking is the best place to start. And so it was for Caroline. This was the prescription to treat her body well. The payoff was great because the pieces of her health were falling into place, and the weight was falling off her body. If you do not exercise at all, the idea is not to start with an expectation that you'll be running a marathon. Just start with a few steps out the door.

## SYMPTOMS

Caroline's problem was common for me to see in many of my clients in their 40s and 50s: weight loss resistance. This occurs when you are trying all the standard ways that you have in the past to lose weight but they are no longer working. Unlike Caroline, you may even be eating healthy (to be determined) and exercising (possibly too much?), yet you are unable to lose pounds. Symptoms of weight loss resistance include:

- Abnormal metabolism, body composition, bone density and mass
- Belly fat
- Bloat
- Constant stress
- Fatigue
- Frustrated
- Irritability or anxiety
- Miserable
- Moody or low mood
- Poor self-esteem
- Social isolation
- Sugar cravings
- Trouble sleeping

Do you identify with any of these?

If you have been trying to lose weight and have been unable to, there are a variety of possibilities for what is standing in the way of your success. For example, you may think you're eating healthy but you really are not (see the Fix Its for guidance), or you may know what to eat but are overeating healthy foods (maybe you're not eating a balanced proportion of fat, fiber, and protein; I'll discuss below). Or maybe your diet is on point but your thyroid isn't producing sufficient hormones (T3 and T4), resulting in a slowed metabolism. Low progesterone or other low hormone levels can also impact your ability to lose weight.

Would you ever think that you need to eat more to lose weight? If you are drastically reducing calories and still not losing, pay attention to this: When you try to cut calories and eat significantly less than what your body needs, your body reacts by reverting to survival mode. In doing so, it literally holds onto all the weight it possibly can. This cycle of not eating enough may have your body fighting for survival. If you feed it less than it needs to operate functionally, it holds on to its fat stores to protect against starvation. A hormonal response occurs—your metabolism slows down to support the body's need to survive.

I've raised the topic of inflammation throughout this book, and it is clear that inflammation lies at the crux of it all. It can cause its own trouble or trigger or exacerbate a hormone response (like when it pushes you into "starvation mode"). When you eat something that is irritating to your system, or to which you are sensitive, a cascade of breakdown begins at the cellular level. Consider as well how inflammation can occur in your body via other harmful ways, for example through your skin or inhalation (I'll talk about toxins later in this chapter). I will show you how to reverse that trend and how good food is essential in your journey towards losing weight.

As you can see, there are many factors involved in weight gain and resistance to weight loss. Understanding how they work can help you learn how to manage your weight more successfully and rid yourself of the extra pounds that plague you. Let's see in more detail what might be going on in your system.

# INFLAMMATION AND WEIGHT LOSS RESISTANCE

The fact that inflammation can inhibit weight loss may not be intuitive, but it is very real. While genetics and environmental factors certainly play a role in the formation of illness or in your struggle to lose weight, inflammation can be even more influential than either of these other factors. You probably think of inflammation as something that happens when you get a bug bite, a splinter, or the flu, or if you sprain your ankle or skin your knee. It turns an injury site red, swollen, hot, and painful. This is your immune system in action, defending you against the threat of infection.

But there is another kind of inflammation that is just as real but much less visible. This is the chronic inflammation that can occur on the inside of your body—in your gut lining, in your blood vessels, and in your internal organs and glands; essentially, in your cells. Chronic inflammation persists after the threat is gone, or is an overreaction by your immune system to something that is not a legitimate threat (like your thyroid gland, or gluten proteins), and it has multiple downstream effects on the systems that regulate your metabolism and your weight. One of the most influential is blood sugar/insulin balance.

## BLOOD SUGAR/INSULIN BALANCE

Once food has been broken down and makes its way into the bloodstream in the form of glucose, the hormone insulin (secreted by your pancreas) escorts the glucose from the blood to the cells that need it to make energy. Normally, human bodies are very good at keeping the level of glucose in the blood at a relatively steady level by secreting insulin in just the right amounts to show glucose the way into the cells. However, when there is an excessive amount of glucose entering the cells by eating overly refined carbohydrates, or eating giant meals, the pancreas starts secreting more insulin to let the body know: *Hey, there's more energy coming. No need to burn any fat. You need to store it!* Excess glucose gets stored in the liver and skeletal muscles to be accessed for energy when the body later needs it, or converted into fat (triglycerides) and stored in adipose tissue (fat cells). In other words, too much glucose in the blood ultimately means too much fat in the cells. The glucose that is stored in the fat cells is more difficult to access, and thus harder to move. This is because it takes more time to break down the adipose tissue and get the glucose out of it. The result can be weight gain, or the dreaded weight loss resistance.

When there is too much insulin in the bloodstream too often, the cells can become insulin resistant, refusing to let in glucose. When this happens, the glucose starts to back up in the bloodstream, causing high blood sugar. This may be reflected as high triglycerides on a lab test, which is often an indicator that someone is eating too many carbs and is at a risk for developing prediabetes or diabetes. The second thing that can happen is called metabolic syndrome. Metabolic syndrome is a collection of symptoms. In women, it causes high estrogen and high testosterone; e.g., weight gain, hair loss, and irritability. In men, it causes high estrogen and low testosterone; e.g., man boobs, beer belly, and low energy. To add insult to injury, that added fat manufactures its own estrogen, acting like an endocrine gland, which causes even more weight gain (I discussed this in more detail in Chapter 5).

Excess adipose tissue = weight gain = inflammation. Monitor your blood sugar for several days (see Chapter 5 to learn how) to get on top of your blood sugar balance. Fortunately, there's a ticket off this roller coaster ride (See the Fix Its in this chapter.).

## DIABETES

Carbs, carbs, and more carbs. No wonder there's a diabetes epidemic in this country![104] Our bodies were not meant to handle so many carbs, especially the refined ones, which can make blood sugar go up and down all day long like an endless roller coaster. The problem is, when this roller coaster of blood sugar happens too regularly, the body gets wise and predicts that you're going to keep the carbs coming in. It pre-generates higher amounts of insulin, often more than what you need, and a few things can happen: 1. The excess insulin sends your blood sugar plummeting, making you crave sugar like it's an emergency. 2. Excess insulin might cause what's known as reactive hypoglycemia (reactive because the body is producing too much insulin in reaction to high blood sugar). The insulin drives the glucose down too low, resulting in a hypoglycemic state. Since 30 to 40% of your brain function is derived from the glucose in your blood, if the level goes beneath its baseline, the brain is not getting fed and has problems. You're in a state of brain fog, irritability, and tiredness; you can't concentrate; and your memory is off. And finally, 3. The presence of insulin in your bloodstream prevents you from burning your fat, and actually keeps you storing pretty much everything you eat as even more fat.

## HUMAN GROWTH HORMONE

Now let's look at some hormones that are also playing a part in weight loss resistance. First up: Human growth hormone (HGH). HGH has an important role in metabolism, as it is the main hormone responsible for breaking down and burning fat. It is produced in the pituitary gland while you sleep. After it's secreted, it travels to the liver and is converted there into growth factors, such as insulin-like growth factor-1 (IGF-1), which is responsible for anabolic benefits, meaning it builds up organs, tissues, and bones. IGF-1 also stimulates lipolysis, which is the breakdown of lipids and fats (goals!) and stimulates protein synthesis.

Considered the anti-aging hormone, HGH is essentially regenerative. It maintains healthy body tissue and preserves the proteins in your hair, nails, skin, collagen, tendons, ligaments, and bones. It promotes repair and restoration of muscle and skeletal growth, retains calcium, and positively influences your cognitive function. HGH begins to decline in your 30s and takes a nosedive in your 50s, which is part of the reason why so many women notice dramatic changes in aging when they hit 50. (Like, *What the heck happened to my skin, and where did I get this belly?*).

There are some nutrients that support HGH production. Vitamin C and dietary fiber are strongly associated with supporting the production of HGH[105] as are the amino acids L-arginine and L-glutamine. On the flip side, alcohol suppresses the release of HGH while you sleep. According to one study, HGH levels dropped up to 75% in adults who had one alcoholic drink.[106] Yikes. Other factors that can cause a decrease in HGH are insomnia, sugar, stress, and excess body weight.

A deficiency can be characterized by:

- Abnormalities in metabolism
- Anxiety
- Body composition and fat masses
- Bone density and mass
- Low mood
- Poor self-esteem
- Social isolation

The number one factor that stimulates HGH production is sleep (see Chapter 4 for sleep tips). See the Fix Its for more ways to boost your HGH.

## LEPTIN & GHRELIN

Leptin and ghrelin are two other hormones directly related to weight gain and loss because they work as a checks and balances system to manage hunger and fullness. Leptin tells the brain to curb the appetite after eating. It's an important part of appetite suppression. It is made by adipose tissue (fat) and secreted into the circulatory system, where it travels to the hypothalamus, telling it, "We have enough fat, so eat less or stop eating." You would think that when you get excess fat on board, that would mean leptin would tell you to cool it on the cupcakes, but unfortunately, we aren't very good at listening to our internal cues, and when we ignore leptin's quiet pleas to cut back for too long, we can become leptin resistant. The fat can be producing leptin but the brain isn't listening so there is no corresponding drop in appetite, and no increased metabolism. Among other things, fructose seems to induce leptin resistance—one of many reasons to avoid high-fructose corn syrup like the plague!

On the other side of the appetite coin is ghrelin, the hunger hormone. When the brain senses that the body needs food, it releases ghrelin, which stimulates appetite, naturally making you want to eat more. Ghrelin also promotes fat storage. When you don't get enough sleep or have low serotonin (or both), your ghrelin level will go up. Have you ever noticed insatiable carb cravings on those days you don't get enough sleep? Blame ghrelin, which can also cause people who are depressed to have strong food cravings and weight gain.

## THE THYROID AND METABOLISM

Remember that the thyroid gland has a huge impact on health and metabolism and it affects every cell in the body. The hormones T3 and T4 (not as sexy sounding as human growth hormone, yet incredibly significant) regulate appetite, energy levels, sleep, sex drive, and overall psychological health. When the thyroid is underactive, everything it regulates slows down. Metabolism slows down. Energy slows down. A lack of activity induces depression and anxiety, which can lead to irritability and what else? Weight gain.

While the gland itself may be an underlying issue to an under-producing thyroid, factors that inhibit the proper production of thyroid hormones include:

- Autoimmune diseases: Celiac disease, Hashimoto's thyroiditis
- Fluoride (antagonist to iodine)
- Infection, trauma, radiation, medications
- Stress
- Toxins: pesticides, mercury, cadmium, lead
- Important nutrients to the health of the thyroid include:
- Iodine
- Iron (foods listed in Chapter 4)
- Selenium
- Tyrosine
- Zinc
- Vitamins B2, B3, B6, C, D, E
- (See associated foods in this chapter under What to Eat.)

The delivery process of T3 to the cells is important to understand. T3 is the most active form of thyroid hormone and is required by every cell in the body to drive cellular metabolism. T4 must be converted into T3 for use by the cells. Whereas T3 is the gas pedal for metabolism, reverse T3, the inactive form, slows metabolism—it hits the brakes. Approximately 20% of T4 is converted into the inactive reverse T3 (rT3), and we want this. We don't want our metabolism just running and running, so rT3 is necessary. However, the problem arises when the conversion of T4 to rT3 increases and metabolism slows. Here are several factors that can cause this situation and the resulting weight gain:

- Certain medications
- Infections
- Inflammation

- Liver/kidney dysfunction

- Low-calorie diet

- Stress

- Toxins

- Trauma

The theme of this book, of course, is that everything you do—what you eat, how you act and respond to the events of your life, and how you interact with the world around you—all have a very real impact on how your body and its most important messengers, your hormones, behave. Are you manifesting a Hormonious life or are you serving yourself up a side dish of symptoms? In this context, it's essential that you consider what the inputs have been (and continue to be). A review of Chapter 2 and its Fix Its may be helpful at this juncture. For example, your struggles with weight could be due to insufficient levels of stomach acid or digestive enzymes. Sounds simple enough yet food that isn't breaking down properly not only slows the system forcing it to work harder but can trigger an imbalance of hormones, resulting in weight that won't budge. Keep using your FTP to help you tease it all out as your life progresses and your circumstances change. When it comes to weight gain or weight loss resistance, the ovaries, adrenal glands, and thyroid gland (sometimes referred to as OAT) are all suspect. You may recall your body's system is a complex arrangement of organs, glands, and communication networks, and the Fix Its throughout this book are designed to help you get to whatever "there" you're aiming for—again, they may overlap, but this is due to the way all the systems in the body interact.

## INTERMITTENT FASTING: SHOULD YOU DO IT FOR WEIGHT LOSS?

Intermittent fasting (IF) or reduced meal frequency is not a new concept, yet it has been a controversial one, especially for women. In an effort to lose weight, some go on starvation or super low-calorie diets that disrupt their systems (especially their hormone and blood sugar balance), to a negative and possibly damaging extent. They may think they are doing intermittent fasting, but this kind of extreme eating is not the same as intermittent fasting. Intermittent fasting just means that you allow your body to go for certain extended periods of time without eating anything so it can focus on repair and rejuvenation while it is not having to digest anything. Typically, this is the time between the end of dinner and the beginning of breakfast. Consider that if you eat your meals at typical times during the day—for example, breakfast in the morning, lunch at noon, and dinner prior to 8 p.m.—you are already living an IF lifestyle (particularly if you don't snack!). While you sleep (and are not eating), your body and cells are in repair-and-rejuvenate mode.

What differentiates the conventional breakfast-lunch-dinner standard of eating to IF or even a starvation diet is that IF outlines a more limited schedule of eating. Some people may eat only between 10 a.m. and 6 p.m., for example, and then fast from 6 p.m. to 10 a.m. the next day. Some make their eating window even shorter, but they still get all the necessary calories and nutrients they need during the period of eating. This is why it is not a starvation diet! It's about timing, not calories. Letting your body rest from digestion can yield a number of health benefits, including weight loss. A number of studies support its effectiveness.

For example, research has shown that IF can improve brain function, including preserving learning and memory. Intermittent fasting has also been shown to improve the cardiovascular system and biomarkers of disease, as well as reduce oxidative stress.[107,108]The California-based company ProLon offers a kit of calorie-restricted meals to be eaten over a period of five days each month for three months. Known as the Fasting Mimicking Diet (FMD), it is scientifically and clinically tested, and its purpose is to induce the body's natural protective and regenerative capabilities.[109]

A variety of methods for practicing intermittent fasting have surfaced over the years, such as eating freely six days a week and not eating on the seventh day, or only eating between noon and 6 p.m. each day. One recent study had participants change their breakfast to 90 minutes later and their dinner to 90 minutes earlier. Findings indicated that those who changed their mealtimes lost, on average, more than twice the body fat than those in the control group.[110] For some, doing a controlled and limited IF can be a great way to jumpstart weight loss efforts while reaping other health benefits, including reducing total body fat, lowering blood pressure, and decreasing the hormone insulin-like growth factor, IGF-1(IGF-1 has been implicated in aging and disease). If you do end up reducing calorie intake, this can provide an opportunity to evaluate your typical way of eating, including reaching for snacks that may be interfering with your diet goals.

Please consult your health care provider if you are interested in doing an IF diet to ensure that doing so will not interfere with your health challenges. IF diets are not recommended for you if your chronic symptoms are in the realm of extreme stress, fatigue, or mood imbalance. They are also not recommended for those with certain metabolic disorders, those who have been diagnosed with a serious medical condition or disease, and those with Diabetes (type 1 and type 2), cardiovascular disease, or cancer unless approved by a healthcare professional. They are also not a good idea for anyone with an eating disorder.

## TOXINS AND WEIGHT GAIN: CAN PLASTIC MAKE YOU FAT?

You know that food plays an essential role in helping you heal and feel better. But what are toxins doing to your weight? They're everywhere—environmental contaminants and chemical endocrine disruptors[111] are challenging your biology, straining your organs to work harder, and adding stress to your interior. Specifically, endocrine disruptors mimic the identity and actions of hormones in the body interfering with their production and stealing receptor sites. Your hormones, and your thyroid in particular, are impacted, and your health is paying the price by causing weight loss resistance.

Over 85,000 chemicals are registered for protection under the U.S. Toxic Substances Control Act (TSCA), the majority of which were grandfathered in with little or no health and safety testing. Science estimates that a newborn baby is born with over 200 toxins right out of the womb. But chemicals aren't the only problem. Other toxins that can affect your health and weight include food additives, antibiotic- and hormone-treated food, toxic bacteria, pollutants, plasticizers, and heavy metals.

Exposure generally occurs through ingestion or inhalation, but skin absorbs toxins as well, meaning anything you put on your skin goes into your body. Sadly, the contents of your makeup drawer can be toxic. Here are some of what you're dealing with every single day when you breathe air, drink water, eat food, clean your body, clean your house, maintain your lawn, and go about all the other tasks of daily living:

- PCBs (polychlorinated biphenyl from fish consumption), BPA (bisphenol A from plastics and canned foods), and PBDEs (Polybrominated diphenyl ethers from flame retardants in mattresses and furniture) all bind to thyroid receptors, so you can't absorb your own thyroid hormones.

- BPA is a synthetic estrogen also referred to as a xenoestrogen that can raise TBG (thyroid binding globulin) levels and mess with your estrogen levels. BPA and phthalates (commonly found in fragrances, plastics, and makeup) are linked to diabetes, insulin resistance, and obesity, and parabens (often found in makeup and personal care products) are linked to low thyroid hormone levels. Phthalates are also linked to low sperm count.[112] Consider the men in your life too!

- Perfluorinated chemicals are found in non-stick cook-ware and food packaging. Exposure is linked to repro-ductive toxicity and thyroid disruption.

- Pesticides and herbicides are linked to gut dysbiosis, endocrine disruption, obesity, and insulin resistance; glyphosate can wreak havoc on the gut, killing healthy gut flora and causing gut hyperpermeability (leaky gut). Non-GMO soy only is recommended; 93% of soy grown in the US is genetically modified. Ditto with corn.

- Heavy metals like lead[113] and cadmium inhibit the conver-sion of T4 to T3 and damage the thyroid gland directly.

If you're not considering toxin exposure in your weight gain equation, you're missing out on a meaningful contributing factor.

## FIX IT

Changing your food habits is hard. For some it's almost the hard-est thing they ever have to do. Food is emotional. Food can feel spiritual. It is part of your childhood and growing up, your culture and your relationships. Holidays and birthdays are opportunities to celebrate and enjoy the foods that connect you to your families and yourself. These things do not necessarily have to change. What matters is what you do on most days when it is not a holiday or a birthday. Consistent good habits on most days accumulate for good results over time.

This is an opportunity for you to finally break free of the pat-terns that may have haunted you and brought you to a place of frustration. Your way hasn't been working. This is your opportu-nity to experiment with a new way of eating. I believe that you have it in you to make the changes to get to better health. These steps are extremely important for your success, so let's keep going! Please keep in mind that food is not the only factor when it comes to weight gain or weight loss resistance. Lifestyle and the environment can largely influence your weight.

## What to Do

### *Evaluate your diet honestly.*

Strive to make everything you eat the best possible nutrient density and quality. For example, try to choose foods that are organic, animal products that are pasture-raised or wild-caught, and in general, foods with as little pesticide, herbicide, and chemical impact as possible. For example, eating grass-fed beef will provide your body with a more balanced profile of omega-3s and omega-6s than feedlot beef. Consider that in addition to the beef you are eating in front of you, you are also ingesting the food that the cow ate as well as any antibiotics and added hormones. If that cow's feed was, for example, genetically modified corn or soy from glyphosate seeds, you're eating that, too.

And remember, every meal and every snack should contain healthy fat, fiber, and protein. Through the process of evaluating your diet honestly, you will continue to calibrate your internal compass. If you take a moment at every meal to assess whether you have included a fat, fiber, and protein, this short pause can eventually become an automatic reminder, even a habit, to add more greens, more healthy fats, and a good solid source of protein every time. Every meal is an opportunity to make a choice that will move your body towards better health. The choice is yours. And it begins at the end of your fork.

## ENVISION YOUR FUTURE SELF

Holding a vision for the way you want your body to look and behave is like creating a mental vision board that reflects your life's vision. Close your eyes and imagine the kind of health you want to achieve. What do you look like? What are you wearing? What are you eating? Six months from now? A year? Five or ten? Create a mission statement to keep yourself on track. If you are swayed by the wafting aroma of the donuts in the office lunchroom or the appetizers being served at your friend's dinner party, by all means, you aren't necessarily forbidden. Life is short and meant to be enjoyed. But for your next food choice, return to your vision and your mission statement. Let them remind you of your calling to better health and energy.

## Increase HGH...

### By exercising.

Exercise increases the production of HGH. Doing short-burst or high-intensity exercises is the best exercise method for increasing HGH.[114]

### By getting good sleep. *(See Chapter 4 for tips.)*

Chronic sleep deprivation causes weight gain by decreasing thyroid output (slowed metabolism), increasing ghrelin (causing hunger), and decreasing HGH. The majority of HGH is released during sleep, so getting good sleep is a priority when it comes to raising your HGH levels.

### By supplementing with L-glutamine.

L-glutamine has been shown to support HGH production.[115]

### By adding in foods to support HGH production

(see the upcoming What to Eat section).

### By laughing more.

Laughter can increase HGH production.[116] One of my favorite things to do is listen to comedians because I love to laugh. Check out apps like Pandora or Laughable on iTunes to spend more time laughing, which gets you a great side dish of HGH. Visit comedy bars or tune into movies or a television series that will get you smiling and laughing out loud.

### Manage your stress.

You already know by now that stress influences you in many ways that can cause you to stress-eat, emotional-eat, or just overeat. Instead of reaching for the cookie or the chips, manage your stress first, in the many ways I talked about in Chapter 3. Getting on top of this body- and life-disruptor can assist in realigning any other imbalances. Sometimes, all it takes is a little bit of solitude and focused breathing to bring down the flames of stress and find your way to calm.

### Honor mealtime + change your relationship with food.

Honoring mealtime and being mindful while eating can support your weight loss efforts.[117] It wasn't until I couldn't eat food for two weeks (SIBO protocol) that I raised my appreciation not only for food itself (I missed chewing, flavors, textures, etc.), but for the process of eating a meal, too. When you take a moment to think about the origins of the foods you're about to eat, participate in the preparation of your meal, and remove distracting variables like TV or computer screens, you are creating a mindful eating experience (see Chapter 2), and ultimately, a connection to the food that is about to feed your cells and nourish your body. Whether you enjoy a meal on your own, or with a friend, taking this thoughtful pause will slow down the eating process, and give you the opportunity to appreciate your meal. This slowdown will also refine your Hormonious compass.

### Upgrade the flavor of your life.

As you consider the role that food has played in your life and as you continue to grow your awareness compass, the trickle-down effect can be profound. Using myself as an example, I have found that it isn't a large leap between eating a particular food, at a particular time, in particular abundance, and recognizing that 1) this is doing my body no good, 2) I can exert control over the situation but I have chosen not to, and 3) I'm eating because I'm nervous, frustrated, upset, disappointed, or fill-in-the-blank. People often use food to fill in emotional holes. Once you hone in on what you're trying to fill, you can start to make plans for alternate ways to satisfy that empty feeling. This is what I mean by Upgrading the Flavor of Your Life.

Review Chapter 5 Fix Its for ideas to add interest, texture, color, sound, and so on into the fabric of your life so that when you are next nervous, fearful, frustrated, disappointed, or fill-in-the-blank, food will not be your first go-to to feel better. Instead, you can look to other sources of activity that can help to dissolve those tensions. Where you put your attention grows. Pay attention to where you pay attention. An imbalance in any direction is an opportunity for you to shift your perspective and create action towards the activities that will satisfy your life itch and fill you up! Then food can return to its original purpose—nourishing your cells, satisfying your palate, and energizing your day.

### *Reduce your exposure to toxic chemicals. Your hormones will thank you.*

**Eat at home more often**. Those who eat out a lot are exposed to more toxins, phthalates in particular.[118] When you prepare your own food, you have direct control over the selection of foods, and know exactly what has been included in its preparation.

**Choose organic** versions of eggs, dairy, meat, fruits and vegetables whenever possible to reduce pesticide, herbicide and other chemical exposures. Ideal meat is grass fed and grass finished. Consult the Environmental Working Group's (EWG) Dirty Dozen guide for fruits and vegetables with the highest and lowest levels of pesticides.

**Eat wild-caught, low mercury** varieties of fish that are smaller, like sardines, which will have lower amounts of mercury than larger ones. Avoid eating farmed salmon due to PCBs, and consult EWG's Consumer Guide to Seafood to stay on top of which fish have the highest levels of mercury. www.nrdc.org/mercury and www.seafoodwatch.org also have information.

**Drink filtered water**. Use a water filtration system and avoid plastic water bottles. Check EWG's Water Filter Guide.

**Review your medicines and supplements** for possible offenders.

**Reduce consumption** of foods and beverages in cans and plastic containers. Purchase canned goods only if they are BPA-free. Avoid touching store receipts which contain BPA residue from the ink and paper.

**Use the EWG's Skin Deep Guide** to cosmetics and Guide to Sunscreens when choosing personal care products. Fragrances contain phthalates; consult skindeep.org to learn more.

**Use glass, ceramic, or stainless-steel** containers for heating and storing food to reduce exposure to phthalates. Also avoid non-stick pots and pans that will contain PCBs.

**Choose fragrance- and solvent-free** detergents and cleaning aids for your home. Consult EWG's Guide to Healthy Cleaning.

**Use integrated pest management** for your home and yard needs. Avoid garden, home and pet pesticides, and fungicides.

Toxic chemicals, endocrine disruptors and environmental pollutants are lurking everywhere. Even minute amounts can be disruptive to your endocrine system and thwart your weight loss efforts. Avoid going into overwhelm by taking a step by step approach. Start with reviewing and considering the food you eat and the water you drink.

Hormonious Tip: Educate yourself about the birth of your food.

It could be a full-time job to learn where and how every food item in your kitchen or meal you plan to eat is grown, harvested, and processed. However, it might be worth your while to select a couple of items that you tend to eat more often—for example, dairy, eggs, or salmon—and do a little more detective work. Your neighborhood supermarket may already have that information, especially if the item is from a local purveyor. If it's not and the information isn't easily available on the packaging, reach out to the company to learn more: in the case of eggs, how are the chickens being raised, what do they eat, are there any added hormones, do they eat non-GMO feed? This exercise not only will give you insight into the process of food production, but it also puts some of the control of what you eat back into your hands. Knowing where your food comes from is another way to strengthen your awareness sense and increase the enjoyment of eating that food.

# WHAT TO EAT

Feed your hormones, balance your blood sugar, increase your HGH, help your body process toxins, and satiate your hunger by making good choices—and the weight *will* start to come off. Here are some strategies:

### Increase foods that support the production of HGH:

- Goji berries are the number one superfood to keep this hormone in check. They contain sesquiterpenoids, which is a natural chemical that helps your body produce HGH. (Please note that goji berries are also a nightshade fruit. Avoid them if you already know you are sensitive to nightshades, and if you aren't sure, pay attention to whether you have any reactions after you eat them. Many people have a sensitivity to this group of foods, which also includes tomatoes, peppers, potatoes, and eggplant.)

- Eating pineapple before bed is helpful for HGH production.

- Algae

- Coconut oil

- Colostrum (available as a protein powder)

- Fava beans

- Gelatin

- Grass fed beef

- Raw cacao

- The amino acid, arginine, is known to secrete HGH as well.[119] The highest amounts will be found in meats.

  o Turkey breast

  o Pork loin

  o Chicken

  o Pumpkin seeds

  o Spirulina

### *Increase leptin.*

Follow these tips to increase the hormone leptin to suppress your appetite.

1. **Eat a protein breakfast.** This is said to increase metabolism by 30%.

2. **Reduce the number of carbs you eat.** Reduce, not exclude. Keep the fiber. Fructose, found in fruit, honey, table sugar, high-fructose corn syrup and agave, seems to induce leptin resistance. Limit accordingly.

3. **Eat slowly, chew well, and stop when you are 80% full.** Don't overeat.

4. **Eat three meals a day.** Only eat snacks if you are experiencing dips in energy and to support balancing your blood sugar. Otherwise, snacks can lead to leptin resistance.

5. **Avoid eating after dinner once in a while.** Leptin is highest in the evening and sets the pattern for nighttime

hormonal regulation and influencing the release of melatonin, thyroid hormone, growth hormone, sex hormones as well as the immune system for proper sleep. Higher levels allow for fat burning during the evening hours where no food is consumed. If you are compelled to eat after dinner, go for a protein which will support melatonin production and sleep.

### *Revamp your relationship with sugar.*

I get it, Sister! Sugar has been in your life for a good, long time, but it's not your friend, it won't take you out on a date, and it's not doing your health any favors. Recall above how it actually tricks you into wanting more? There is nothing good about that. Here are ways to cut your ties with sugar dramatically. These are also found in my free download (http://wellnessgirl.net/hormoniousplan):[120]

1. **Eat balanced meals, aka balance your blood sugar—remember, fiber, protein, and good fat.**

2. **Consider the health of your gut; sugar is a fuel for all types of bad bacteria and candida (yeast).** Eat probiotic-rich foods to ensure a healthy balance (see Chapter 2).

3. **Replace artificial sweeteners that are wreaking havoc on your liver and microbiome.** The less processed and refined, the better.
   - Explore options like raw honey, pure maple syrup, stevia, coconut sugar, and dates (which are fibrous). These can still impact your blood sugar (except stevia) so use sparingly. Some practitioners believe that putting anything sweet (I'm not talking fruits or vegetables) on the tongue can trigger the brain to think *"SUGAR!"* triggering the dopamine pathway and the ramifications of sugar addiction.[121]
   - Other options less known but worth exploring

are lucuma, Yacon syrup, and coconut nectar.

- o Lakanto is a natural sweetener made from monk fruit also known as Luo Han Guo and has a zero glycemic index.
- o Erythritol, also non-glycemic,[122] is an alternative to and contains fewer calories than sugar. It is a sugar alcohol[123] derived from fermenting corn. Though generally recognized as safe (GRAS) by the FDA, some may experience digestive upset and high doses (50 grams) have been shown to cause nausea.[124]

1. **Drink more water.** (Sound familiar?) Often your cravings are masquerading as thirst. Always drink water before you reach for a snack. You may just be dehydrated.

2. **Make breakfast protein-rich and delicious to set the tone and frame your day.**

3. **Snack right to avoid those dips in energy that accompany bad snacks.**
   - o Bean dips such as hummus, with celery, jicama, or spread over romaine leaves
   - o Sliced apple with cinnamon and almond butter: sprinkle bee pollen on top for added protein.
   - o Chia pudding
   - o Bulletproof snack bar
   - o Smashed avocado with salt, lime juice, and sliced carrots

4. **Spice up your snacks and meals.** Cinnamon helps stabilize blood sugar, cayenne pepper promotes weight loss, and ginger supports digestion. Other spices will elevate the flavors that naturally sweeten foods like cardamom, nutmeg, and cloves.

5. **Need a hit of sugar?** Bake a sweet potato and add a pat of grass-fed butter or coconut oil, some cinnamon, and a pinch of sea salt. Incorporate other sweet-tasting vegetables into your meals like spaghetti squash, carrots, spiralized beets, or bell peppers. Fruit is also an option.

6. **Be honest with yourself.** If you can't resist certain items, remove them from your home and don't buy them. You can still indulge every now and then. Aim to do so with quality products, like a couple squares of dark chocolate that are 80% or higher cacao.

7. **Be kind, patient, and forgiving.** Change takes time. The more you pay attention to your food choices and what they're comprised of, the more empowered you will be to continue to make better choices. Change will come, I promise. If you're not willing to make change, accept this, and move on. Do not berate yourself.

### *Compose every meal with fat, fiber, and protein for your metabolic needs.*

Do I keep saying this? That's because it is *so important!* To determine the right proportion for you will take a bit of experimentation. For example, if you are used to eating heavy carb meals, the transition to lower carbs will take time. It's more important to focus on replacing junk food with higher-quality nutrient foods than analyzing the calorie count. The best way to move forward is to always ask yourself these three critical questions after you've eaten. Are you experiencing:

- A sense of satiety?
- Good, solid energy?
- A sense of well-being?

These important questions and the answers you give yourself will help you frame your meals going forward. If you are not feeling satisfied by your meal, consider whether you had enough protein on the plate.

Same with the fat and fiber elements. Did you have enough fat? Maybe you should add more the next meal. Fiber will also provide a feeling of fullness. Consider the portion of fiber-rich carbs in your meal too. If your energy dips and you're tired, evaluate that meal in terms of its fat and fiber content. Did the meal have too many refined or processed foods? This can explain the drop in energy. Your meal should also provide you with a sense of feeling nourished. If your mood sinks or you are feeling off, review your meal for possible offenders again. Keep track by notating in your Every-Day Plan (explained in Chapter 7).

Next, I'll provide you with some basic 'recipe' options to give you a sense of what is meant by fat, fiber, and protein. For every meal that you have, is there a protein (animal, plant-based, etc.)? Is there a fiber (the possibilities are many and the following list is just a small representation)? Is there a healthy fat?

## YOUR BODY NEEDS PROTEIN

Too little protein combined with too many carbs can result in weight gain.[125] Protein is comprised of amino acids, the building blocks of life. They are essential for our muscles, skin, hair, and bones. Your hormones, neurotransmitters, DNA and most of your muscles are made from amino acids, and protein is needed for your tissues, blood oxygenation and basic cell activity.

- Animal proteins are considered 'complete' because they contain all the amino acids your body requires from food, known as the essential amino acids. Best choices are pasture-fed, free-range and organic. Wild-caught fish are an excellent source of omega-3 fatty acids. Farm-raised fish are typically low in omega-3s due to a diet devoid of aquatic plants. They have higher levels of PCBs, are fed with corn or soy pellets (which contain pesticide residues), are routinely dosed with antibiotics, and are given synthetic dyes to make their flesh pink. If you eat farm-raised, get to know that farm, what those fish are eating, and how they are maintained. Animal proteins include:

- o   Eggs
- o   Fish
- o   Meat
- o   Poultry
- o   Shellfish

- Plant proteins are considered 'incomplete' because they don't contain all essential amino acids. High protein vegetables include:

  - o   Asparagus
  - o   Bok choy
  - o   Broccoli
  - o   Brussel sprouts
  - o   Cauliflower
  - o   Dark leafy greens (collard greens, spinach, mustard greens, etc.)
  - o   Tofu, tempeh and spirulina are also plant proteins

- Protein powders can be a great way to get protein into your diet by way of a smoothie. Protein powders are made from either:

  - o   Animal protein (whey, casein, collagen, beef or eggs), or
  - o   Plant protein (soy, rice, pea, hemp or sprouted grains)

- Beans and legumes are good sources of both protein and carbs. They also contain vitamins and minerals like Vitamin B9 (folate), potassium, iron and magnesium.

- Dairy products like milk and yogurt are good sources of protein and carbs, provided that you tolerate them well. If you choose to consume dairy, make sure you opt for organic sources. Non-organic options will have hormones and other undesirable elements.

- Nuts and seeds contain both protein and fat. They also contain other vitamins and minerals like magnesium, zinc, selenium and copper.

## EAT QUALITY FATS

Fat is an important source of energy for the body, helping to heat the body, drive metabolic processes, and move muscles. Fat is also necessary for brain health, connective tissue, your digestive system and enhances hormone and neurotransmitter cell communication. It's your friend because it provides a feeling of satiety. If you've eaten a meal sans fat, and are hungry soon after, that should provide you with valuable information. The healthiest sources of fat are those that are monounsaturated.

Sources include:

- Avocado oil
- Avocados
- Olive oil
- Olives
- Red meat
- Various nuts and seeds
- Whole milk

Saturated fat is also acceptable and considered a good fat. It is also very stable, so it's good for cooking. The same quality requirements apply here. Sources should be organic, pasture-raised and without any added hormones, antibiotics, chemicals, etc.:

- Butter
- Cocoa butter
- Coconut oil
- Egg yolk
- Ghee (clarified butter)
- MCT oil
- Meat fat
- Palm kernel oil
- Palm oil (from sustainable sources)

**Hormonious Tip:** MCT oils (medium-chain triglycerides) are a form of saturated fatty acids that have numerous benefits, including improving the health of those with fat malabsorption issues and improving hormone levels and mood. They are also recognized for improving energy levels and cognition (bye-bye, brain fog!). They contain antioxidant properties and are capable of combating harmful bacteria, viruses, fungi, and parasites.

MCTs are particularly beneficial because of their ability to be taken up directly by the intestines into circulation therefore bypassing physiological steps required for fat intake, and the capacity to be metabolized into usable forms of energy like glucose.[126]

Coconut oil and palm kernel oil are both MCT oils, but MCT oils that contain higher levels of caprylic and capric acids are more desirable for improving numerous health problems. For weight loss purposes, using oils with these higher levels can lead to a greater rate of weight loss than using olive oil.[127] You can find them in the health food store.

**Hormonious Tip:** How you store your oils to preserve their integrity is important. For example, polyunsaturated oils such as flaxseed oil, in particular, cannot be stored at room temperature and must be kept in light protective, opaque containers. Monounsaturated oils, such as olive oil, do not need to be refrigerated.

Take care in how you heat oils. Some oils are better at higher heat, while others can degrade at high temperatures making their use ill-advised—beneficial nutrients are lost, and degraded oils can impart free radicals and oxidative stress. These are the preferred cooking techniques for a sample of oils:[128]

| High-heat cooking | Medium-heat cooking (200 to 300 degrees) | Low-heat cooking |
|---|---|---|
| Coconut | Olive | Almond |
| Peanut* | Corn* | Sesame |
| High oleic safflower | Hazelnut | Sunflower butter |
| Avocado | | |
| Red palm | | |

*Critical to use organic because of high-pesticide use.

## OMEGAS

**Omega-3**'s we can only get from food. They're important for brain health, development and reducing inflammation. Fatty fish is an excellent source.

• Chia seeds

- Flaxseeds and flaxseed oil
- Herring
- Mackerel
- Oysters
- Salmon
- Sardines
- Soybeans (organic only)
- Walnuts

**Omega-6** fatty acids are abundant in Western diets as discussed previously. Avoid processed vegetable oils like corn and soybean oil, as well as fried foods, and aim to balance with omega-3s. Omega-6s are also found in nuts and seeds:

- Almonds
- Cashews
- Walnuts
- Sunflower seeds

## CHOOSE YOUR CARBS WISELY

Some carbs offer more nutrient density than others. The best sources will provide you energy, vitamins, minerals, and phytonutrients—all of which are important to brain function, digestive health, and your hormones (see Chapter 5 for further discussion on carbs). Consider the following sources:

- Include a variety of vegetables—both starchy and non-starchy. Those that are high in fiber will help stabilize your blood sugar and keep you full longer.

- Though many fruits are high in carbs because of the natural sugars found in them, they also offer vitamins, minerals, and phytonutrients.

- Limit amounts, but reach for fruit in place of refined sweet foods that deplete you.

- Whole grains that are unprocessed are high in fiber, slow to digest, and full of vitamins and minerals. Processed ones are the opposite.

- Beans and legumes can be good sources of carbs and proteins if you tolerate them. They contain vitamins and minerals, like Vitamin B9 (folate), potassium, iron, and magnesium.

- Dairy products like milk, yogurt, and cheese are good sources of both carbs and proteins, provided that you can tolerate them. They do offer the body vitamins and minerals but are not necessary to include for a balanced diet. If you choose to eat dairy, full-fat and organic sources are recommended.

## A KALEIDOSCOPE OF NUTRIENTS

Choose a kaleidoscope of color so that you can experience the benefits that each hue provides.

*RED*
Eat reds for the following beneficial properties: anti-cancer, anti-inflammatory, cell protection, gastrointestinal health, heart health, hormone health, and liver health.

- Apples
- Beans (adzuki, kidney, red)
- Beets

- Bell peppers
- Blood oranges
- Cranberries
- Cherries
- Grapefruit (pink)
- Goji berries
- Grapes
- Onions
- Plums
- Pomegranate
- Potatoes
- Radicchio
- Radishes
- Raspberries
- Strawberries
- Sweet red peppers
- Rhubarb
- Rooibos tea
- Tomatoes
- Watermelon

### *ORANGE*

Orange for: anti-cancer, anti-bacterial, immune health, cell protection, reduced mortality, reproductive health, skin health, and a source of Vitamin A.

- Apricots
- Bell peppers

- Cantaloupe

- Carrots

- Mangoes

- Nectarines

- Oranges

- Papaya

- Persimmons

- Pumpkin

- Squash (acorn, buttercup, butternut, winter)

- Sweet potatoes

- Tangerines

- Turmeric root

- Yams

### *YELLOW*

Yellow for: anti-cancer, anti-inflammatory, cell protection, cognition, eye health, heart health, skin health, and vascular health.

- Apples

- Asian pears

- Bananas

- Bell peppers

- Corn, corn-on-the-cob

- Ginger root

- Lemon

- Millet

- Pineapple

- Starfruit

- Succotash
- Summer squash

## *GREEN*

Green for: anti-cancer, anti-inflammatory, brain health, cell protection, skin health, hormone balance, heart health, and liver health.

- Apples
- Artichoke
- Asparagus
- Avocado
- Bamboo sprouts
- Bean sprouts
- Bell peppers
- Bitter melon
- Bok choy
- Broccoli
- Broccolini
- Brussels sprouts
- Cabbage
- Celery
- Cucumbers
- Edamame/Soy beans (Organic)
- Green beans
- Green peas
- Green tea/matcha (organic only)
- Greens (arugula, beet, chard/swiss chard, collard, dandelion, kale, lettuce, mustard, spinach, turnip)

- Limes
- Okra
- Olives
- Pears
- Snow peas
- Watercress
- Zucchini

### *BLUE/PURPLE/BLACK*

Eat blue for these beneficial properties: anti-cancer, anti-inflammation, cell protection, cognitive health, heart health, and liver health.

- Bell peppers
- Berries (blue, black, boysenberries, huckleberries, marionberries)
- Cabbage
- Carrots
- Cauliflower
- Eggplant
- Figs
- Grapes
- Kale
- Olives
- Plums
- Potatoes
- Prunes
- Raisins
- Rice (black or purple)

## *WHITE/TAN/BROWN*

Eat white/tan/brown for: anti-cancer, anti-microbial, cell protection, gastrointestinal health, heart health, hormone health, and liver health.

- Apples
- Applesauce
- Bean dips
- Cauliflower
- Cocoa
- Coconut
- Coffee
- Dates
- Garlic
- Ginger
- Jicama
- Legumes (chickpeas, beans or peas, hummus, lentils, peanuts)
- Mushrooms
- Nuts (almonds, cashews, pecans, walnuts)
- Onions
- Pears
- Sauerkraut
- Seeds (flax, hemp, pumpkin, sesame, sunflower)
- Shallots
- Soy (organic only)
- Tahini
- Tea (black, white)

- Whole grains (brown rice, oat, quinoa)

# EAT YOUR VITAMINS AND MINERALS.

- Vitamin A

    **Vitamin A** is essential to your vision, immune function, bone development and more. It's also required for detoxification of certain chemicals and is essential to the health of your epithelial tissue, which lines your gut and glands throughout your body.

    o Bell peppers

    o Bok choy

    o Cantaloupe

    o Carrots

    o Dark leafy greens (collard greens, kale, spinach, Swiss chard, etc.)

    o Egg yolks

    o Fish liver

    o Grass-fed butter

    o Liver

    o Organic whole milk

    o Sweet potatoes

    o Tropical fruits

- Vitamin E

    **Vitamin E** is a fat-soluble vitamin that provides antioxidant protection and supports cognition and brain health plus eye health and immune system function.

    o Almonds

    o Asparagus

- o Avocado
- o Dark leafy greens (beet greens, mustard greens, spinach, Swiss chard, turnip greens, etc.)
- o Sunflower seeds
- Vitamin K

**Vitamin K** is required for bone development, cardiovascular health, cellular function and soft tissue integrity (prevents calcification).

- o Asparagus
- o Broccoli
- o Bok choy
- o Brussels sprouts
- o Cabbage
- o Cauliflower
- o Dark leafy greens (beet greens, collard greens, kale, mustard greens, spinach, Swiss chard, turnip greens, etc.)
- o Parsley
- Copper

This trace mineral provides antioxidant protection, supports cell/tissue growth and repair, balances your cholesterol and supports energy production and nervous system health.

- o Apricots (dried)
- o Asparagus
- o Dark chocolate
- o Dark leafy greens
- o Lentils
- o Liver (beef)
- o Mushrooms

- o   Nuts
- o   Seeds
- o   Shrimp
- Iodine

**Iodine** is essential to thyroid health and hormone production, metabolism, and cellular energy.

- o   Cod
- o   Cow milk
- o   Eggs
- o   Salmon, sardines, scallops, shrimp, tuna
- o   Sea vegetables
- o   Strawberries
- Manganese

**Manganese** provides antioxidant support, blood sugar control, and supports bone, skin, hair, and nail health.

- o   Beans
- o   Cinnamon
- o   Cloves
- o   Dark leafy greens (collard greens, kale, spinach, Swiss chard, etc.)
- o   Oats
- o   Pineapple
- o   Rice (brown)
- o   Seeds
- o   Turmeric
- Molybdenum

**Molybdenum** is a trace mineral that supports metabolism and enzyme production.

- o   Barley (contains gluten)

- o Beans
- o Lentils
- o Oats
- o Peas
- Selenium

**Selenium** is important to thyroid and heart health. It also provides antioxidant protection and supports your immune system.

- o Asparagus
- o Beef
- o Brazil nuts (amount depends on quality of soil)
- o Clams
- o Cod
- o Mushrooms
- o Organ meats (liver, kidney)
- o Oysters
- o Poultry
- o Salmon, sardines, tuna
- o Shrimp
- o Tofu (organic only)
- Sulphur

**Sulphur** is a major mineral that supports metabolism, insulin production, and helps control inflammation and pain. It also contributes to the health of your skin, hair, and nails.

- o Beans
- o Eggs
- o Fish
- o Meats
- o Milk
- o Nuts

       o   Poultry
- Zinc

**Zinc** is a trace mineral that your body needs in small amounts. It supports your metabolism (ding, ding, ding!), as well as immune system function and skin health. It is important for sensory organ health, such as taste and vision. Though highly concentrated in whole grains, legumes, and nuts, zinc is not as absorbable due to its binding of phytic acid from these sources. Zinc can also help lower excess cortisol (are you stressed out?) and is a co-factor to produce calming neurotransmitters like serotonin and GABA. Even more, it is needed to make testosterone. Eat your zinc!

       o   Ginger root

       o   Meat and poultry (ground round steak, lamb chops, beef liver, egg yolk, chicken)

       o   Fresh oysters (contain highest levels of zinc)

       o   Seafood (sardines, anchovies, tuna, haddock)

       o   Shellfish (clams, shrimp, crab, lobsters, and mussels)

       o   Vegetables, like asparagus, green peas, parsley, mushrooms, spinach depending on soil condition

## WHAT NOT TO EAT

Remove the following foods for a period of 30 days:

- Alcohol

- Artificial sweeteners

- Dairy (Many individuals may have a dairy sensitivity and not make the connection between symptoms and dairy, so it's worth giving this a try, even if it means a temporary cheese hiatus!)

- Gluten (the protein in wheat, rye, barley, and conventional oats); see page 57 for more gluten-based foods.

- Refined and overly processed foods (anything in a package with more than three ingredients, and anything made with white flour and/or white sugar and/or trans fats and/or vegetable oils other than cold-pressed olive, coconut, and nut oils)

- Sugar (which includes white sugar and all refined or processed sweeteners)

- Any food to which you already know you are sensitive

Giving yourself this 30-day time frame will help you suss out what is aggravating your symptoms and provide a baseline from which to go forward. Doing this can bring forth dietary clarity and some pretty dramatic symptom relief. After 30 days, assess how you feel and whether the removal of these items has made a difference in your health and wellness and/or improved your efforts to lose weight. If you would like to add an item that you removed back into your diet, do so by adding that item on its own. For example, add back gluten-containing foods over a period of several days before adding back any other foods that you removed. This way you can clearly associate any recurrence of reactions or symptoms with that specific food. If you don't have any reactions, that food may be okay for you. Utilize the EveryDay Plan (found at wellness-girl.net/hormoniousplan and explained in Chapter 7) to help you stay organized and keep track of foods and symptoms.

If you continue to have symptoms at the end of 30 days, consult with an FM practitioner[129] to consider doing an Elimination Diet, or to conduct food sensitivity testing. The list below represents other foods that you may have a sensitivity to or be intolerant of.

- Other inflammatory foods that people often remove include:
  - o Caffeine

- o  Corn
- o  Eggs
- o  Peanuts
- o  Shellfish
- o  Soy

## WHAT TO TAKE

- Vitamin D

  The fat-soluble sunshine (hormone) vitamin is essential and supports metabolism, blood sugar regulation, immune system function, and so much more. For women, it's particularly important for bone health. Without it, the body can't absorb the calcium it ingests and thus steals it from bones, resulting in osteoporosis or fractures. While the best way to get Vitamin D is through direct sunlight, doing so can prove difficult depending on where you live and the time of year. In the right conditions, getting 10 to 15 minutes a day on your arms and legs a few times a week would be optimal. Note food options on Page 151. Your Vitamin D levels should be obtained regularly and as part of your annual serum labs. Vitamin D3 is best utilized when taken with Vitamin K2.

**Hormonious Tip:** One of the ways that conventional medicine differs from FM is in the analysis of lab results. Conventional medicine looks at the clinical or reference range through the lens of disease diagnosis, whereas FM assesses for a risk before disease develops. This distinction is an important one.

An example:

Vitamin D, 25-hydroxy in units of ng/ml:[130]

Conventional          Functional

32-100                55-80

The functional range is narrower as FM is taking a preventative approach and so recognizes that the body is not functioning optimally. Functional medicine does not wait for a disease state to present itself, rather, it looks for clues and patterns in which you can make changes and tweak your health to prevent a negative outcome. In the example above where the conventional range for Vitamin D (25-hydroxy in units of ng/ml) is 32-100, if your level is at 32, an FM practitioner will encourage you to increase your Vitamin D intake because the FM range is narrower. The ramifications of the low level could be several, the bottom line being that you do not have sufficient Vitamin D in your system to perform important functions—such as optimal metabolism, blood sugar balance, and so on. If you follow the conventional approach, your physician may not make the recommendation to increase your Vitamin D intake—a missed opportunity. This is part of the beauty of FM. The more you know, the more you can control your health for a better outcome.

## MEAL SAMPLES

Here's some inspiration for organizing nutrient-dense, satisfying meals to encourage weight loss.

### [Serves 1] Breakfast

- Two eggs cooked in coconut oil. Place mixed greens, ½ a diced avocado and sliced bell peppers in a grain-free tortilla. Add eggs and 4-5 basil leaves on top. Sprinkle with sea salt and hit with hot sauce for a boost of flavor.

- Smoothie (See Page 123 for recipe ideas)

### Lunch

- Go to Town Turkey Salad.[131] Break apart sliced turkey and add to any mixed greens and arugula, ½ diced avocado, diced beets, chopped red onion and a table-spoon of pumpkin seeds. Sprinkle olive oil, lemon juice and sea salt on top.

- Chunks of cooked salmon atop a gluten-free bagel, lac-tose-free cream cheese or mashed avocado, arugula, and capers along with a side of zucchini slices sautéed in olive oil and seasoned with sea salt and paprika.

## *Dinner*

- Sliced chicken breast, butternut squash spirals cooked in coconut oil, roasted broccoli, and quinoa salad (cooked quinoa that's been cooled; mix with diced cucumbers, tomatoes, purple onion, olive oil, lemon juice, salt and pepper).

- AnyTime Digestive soup (See page 85) with a side of organic white rice (add chopped cilantro to rice and a squeeze of lime; the same can be done for the soup).

## *Snacks*

- Simplify Truffle balls (See page 194)

- Kale chips. Break apart a bunch of kale. Massage with olive oil, sprinkle with sea salt, one teaspoon curry powder (or seasoning of your choice) and one table-spoon nutritional yeast (excellent protein). Bake at 350 degrees for 15 to 20 minutes (time varies based on texture desired).

- Sliced apple with almond butter, cinnamon and bee pollen.

- Blended frozen banana with one tablespoon sunflow-er seed butter, ¼ cup almond milk and one tablespoon cacao nibs.

# CHAPTER 7

## THE MASTERPIECE.
## YOUR BODY,
## YOUR HEALTH.

*"Give yourself the gift of finishing strong."*
*—Marie Forleo*

You are on a journey, and perhaps at a crossroads. If you have been struggling with chronic symptoms (and yet your doctor says you're fine), these are your 'check engine' lights, alerting you that something is going on and that something needs attention on the interior. Throughout this book, I have provided you with a variety of tools to support you in responding to the malfunctions happening at the cellular level and disrupting your balance of hormones. As you make the changes that I propose, please hold the idea at the forefront of your mind that in order to achieve a Hormonious balance, or at least live adjacent to it, your cells require the utmost care, and you carry a very high percentage of control over the inputs. Your ever-developing awareness compass will become a most trusted asset.

Always remember that your path is about the experience, not achieving a perfect balance at all times, as there is no such thing. Instead, show your cells love by honoring your body every day and throughout the day—thoughtful food, mindful breathing, energy-promoting movement, rejuvenating rest, and engaged relationships. Honor your soul with joyful, high vibe activities, and refresh your spirit in nature. You are a masterpiece, and I want to see you shining brightly, energetically, with your exterior reflecting a kick-ass interior. And though this book isn't meant to be a call to action on the health of the environment, the trickle-down effect may occur as you consider the quality of the food you eat, the products you use on your body and in your home, and the impact your health-evoking behavior has on all those around you and those you will one day leave behind.

Go to wellnessgirl.net/hormoniousplan to download your roadmap, the EveryDay Plan. The EveryDay Plan will be your daily navigator and accountability tool to keep you organized and flowing forward—a week on a page gives your health structure, and provides a home for tracking symptoms, food, and mood (in the notes). In time, you may not need this, but for now, use it to guide your days to ensure you're hitting the high notes towards better health. Print it out weekly or fill it out online.

You can find a downloadable copy of the Hormonious Habit Master List (HHML) at the same link above. Though not exhaustive, the HHML provides a list of most Fix It options contained in this book. Note that some Fix Its apply to all categories of chronic issues, and are denoted with an asterisk. Select a Fix It (or more) that you would like to start integrating into your life by circling it and listing it on your EveryDay Plan beneath the 'Week of' reference. Refer to your EveryDay Plan daily (and throughout your day) to ensure that you are taking steps to develop that element into a

Hormonious Habit. It can be a What to Eat, Do, or Take. Check off items that you feel you have incorporated into your life as true habits. Every time you check off an item, you will feel a sense of accomplishment. Keep going...

You'll note that throughout this book, I have provided you with several recipes meant to be foundational as you refine your own diet, meaning that you can add to them and/or make swaps according to your preferences. They are meant to be ultimately adaptable to you and your needs. The download will also include the recipes contained in this book (you're welcome!). Feel free to use any recipe outside of this book as well. You can always apply the core concepts of Hormonious: clean proteins, fats, and fiber, to support your health agenda along with reducing/eliminating your exposure to toxins—all with the aim of allowing your hormones to function optimally. The Hormonious Fundamental Foods List document provides an organized list of foods to inspire meal planning and can also be downloaded at http://wellnessgirl.net/hormoniousplan).

I realize that I have provided you with a lot of information in this book. It is not meant to be done all-at-once today. Or tomorrow. It's meant to be incorporated regularly and periodically so that your new habit(s) become a seamless part of your life. Some habits will take you less time. Others longer. Remember, once a Hormonious habit is firmly ingrained, check it off your Hormonious Habit Master List. Move down to another one. Adopt one weekly until it's fully rooted into your being like brushing your teeth or taking your dog for a walk. If I had to prioritize, I would say that drinking more (filtered) water and eating more vegetables should be at the top of the list, along with stress-reducing activities like daily focused breathing.

## PREPARATION

The best opportunity for success is to be organized. Examine your kitchen and its food contents. The foods that you will start adding into your rotation may not be recognizable or welcome to other family members (old habits die hard). If you are the one making food for the family, you will slowly be tweaking their diet (to their benefit) as well. In the meantime, carve out space for yourself in the fridge and on a shelf that is your clean space—a no-junk zone. Keep those areas designated for yourself (and your partner if they are joining you) and make sure to let your family members know. Donate or throw out foods that no longer serve you or your vision of health.

Feel free to use the 5 Rs of FM to structure your overall health goals (See Chapter 2) especially if you are working with a functional medicine practitioner. Accountability apps like Habit Tracker or HabitShare can keep you aligned with your objectives, or if you prefer one-on-one support, check out the app Coach.me. Graduates of the IIN program can also support you to reach your goals. If you're interested in FM support for lab testing or medical oversight and partnering, visit The Institute for Functional Medicine site. Graduates of Functional Diagnostic Nutrition can also guide you, as well as provide lab testing options, analysis, and direction.

Your FMP is ideal for keeping track of all other facets of your well-being, not only to narrow in on or possibly close the circle on what some of the root causes may have been to your current health state, but also as a point of reference. As you step forward and make changes, you may be crossing off medications, adding supplements, improving your sleep routine, refining your exercise schedule, incorporating breathwork, and so on. You will be examining your relationships, your work satisfaction, and creating a relationship with your 90-year-old self. Remember her? Check in with her every so often so that she can help keep you on track.

Root cause analysis is not just an exercise in evaluating your food choices. It is a pre-birth-to-present survey combined with a step-by-step action plan to elevate and upgrade your life for whole-body health. After all, as the captain of your ship, you have the power to navigate towards your best life possible.

**Hormonious Reflection:** Whole-body health—it's not just about the food. It simply is not enough to eat well. In order to rejigger your body to a state of Hormonious health, incorporate the Fix Its provided throughout to address and upgrade the following lifestyle factors:

- Stress reduction (breathing exercises; tend to personal and work relationships)
- Improve sleep
- Exercise regularly
- Supplement as needed
- Make joyful activities a priority
- Optional: leave the world in a better place

**Hormonious A-ha!** Invest in your health by partnering with a health-care practitioner who cares about your health almost as much as you do. FM has not yet pervaded our over-burdened health care system. What this means for you is that you may not get the full attention, understanding, or direction you need from your current health care professional. But you should. You should demand this or find someone who is willing to go the distance with you, to help guide your process with the goal of discovering the underlying cause(s) of your issues. Allow the commonsense philosophy of FM outlined in Hormonious to frame your health journey going forward. Targeted functional lab testing can light the path. This need not be an expensive endeavor. A knowledgeable FM practitioner can escort you through this process with the understanding that you are doing your part by 1) following the directives set out here (along with any other helpful and/or inspiring resources that can illuminate your way forward); 2) shouldering the responsibility that what you do and don't do matters; and 3) recognizing that achieving good health is not a straight line but a curvy one (so your patience is required). If you cannot find an FM practitioner local to you, check out the Resources for a list of online options, as well as IFM.org or emailing support@afdnp.com for a referral to a Functional Diagnostic Nutrition Practitioner.

The day-to-day of your health is predominantly in your hands, but the process can be made sweeter and more motivating with the support of a wellness guide. Having a trusted health partner as your co-pilot can give you the confidence and motivation to keep going when you hit bumps. Don't underestimate the power of this powerful support system.

This is the kind of investment that will pay off when you need it most. I believe your 90-year-old self would agree.

# EPILOGUE

*"A year from now you will have wished you started today."*
*—Jay Shetty*

While much of who you are is determined by your genes, you are largely a product of the circumstances from which you came, the choices you have made, and the choices you *will* make! Ultimately, how you live can influence the expression of your genes, not just in your past but now and in your future. And while the road that has led you to your current health challenges has probably taken you on some unexpected turns, through circular routes, and perhaps to some dead ends, having the power over your health by exercising your control over your own decisions can become an incredibly influential tool. Much of this influence starts with what's on the end of your fork and continues with your commitment to being present in this and every moment, to breathing through the difficulties, to respecting the potential and limits of your body, and to considering the health of your environment. If you are fortunate enough that your body has not yet reached its tipping point towards disease, then, given the choice between pharma and food, I hope you now see why it makes much more sense to choose the most cost effective, least dangerous, and most you're-the-captain-of your-ship route. I hope you will choose food.

The process of healing can be slow, uncomfortable, and frustrating. But it can also be invigorating, joyful, and life-changing. It can also be little-black-dress happy—the way you feel when you are your sexiest self. Start with right now, this moment, then consciously, deliberately implement small, even tiny, changes day by day—sustainable ones that feel good. Remind yourself that you've got this.

The answers to your health conundrum will take time to suss out. The tweaks you implement in the name of your own well-being won't all happen at once. Continue to dial into what your body is telling you, developing that internal awareness compass. What makes it feel better, and what makes it feel worse? Consider, too, what is motivating your choices. Influences from your past? Your childhood? Current stressors? Toxic relationships? These clues are signposts on your journey and your recognition of them can help you reach your health goals more efficiently.

You have a choice. The state of your health is largely up to you. Vote for an amplified life by aligning your actions with the vision you want and taking step-by-step movements towards a healthier, more Hormonious existence. Accept that it will take time to meet your goals, and that even when you arrive at them and feel amazing, that is not the end, for it is the journey you travel that is delightful and hard and worth it.

Hormonious is what you deserve to feel.

Your future self will thank you.

Truly,

Karen

Wellness Girl

# ACKNOWLEDGMENTS

There are many people who deserve thanks for supporting me on this journey to Hormonious. My parents top the list. Paula and Jacob would be incredibly proud, but also ultra-pleased that my English major in college paid off. My main man, Yossi. Your presence in my life is what made this possible. Thanks is simply not enough to express the deep love and appreciation I feel for you and our life together. My boy tribe—Noah, Rahm & Tai—thank you for your patience, understanding, and willingness to try any and all foods I bring home or create. Thank you also for forgiving me, the imperfect parent.

Sometimes words alone can't express gratitude, yet my path here was supported in great part by learning how to breathe, meditate, and look within. Ramaa Krishnan at Full Bloomed Lotus came into my life when I needed her most. Your teachings are always with me.

Thank you to Joshua Rosenthal, the founder of Institute for Integrative Nutrition, for creating a program that got the ball rolling for me. I don't know where I'd be if I didn't start there. I am so appreciative of Karen Malkin for pointing me to IIN, and providing an example of what it means to be a dedicated health coach and staunch champion of health. I (we) also owe her a large thanks for sharing her truffle recipe on which Simplify is based.

Andrea Nakayama taught me not only about the intersection of where food and physiology meet, but also how an incredibly traumatic event can become the guiding light in your life. Thank you deeply for supporting *Hormonious*.

My expert gurus—Drs. Mark Hyman, David Perlmutter, Trupti Gokani, Terry Wahls, Frank Lipman, Tom O'Bryan, Hyla Cass, Kelly Brogan, Felice Gersh, Aviva Romm, Dan Kalish, Vincent Pedre, Jill Carnahan—these are FM leaders and practitioners who are paving the road on which commonsense medicine can grow and thrive.

I owe Much appreciation to those who believed in me enough to support this writing. I am indebted to you, Drs. Terry Wahl, Trupti Gokani, Felice Gersh, Yehuda Shoenfeld, and James Maskell.

Dr. Andrew Weil—I have to single you out. Your 4-7-8 transformed me and every single person I share it with (who does it consistently!). Thank you for featuring it so prominently in your lectures.

My friends are incredibly important to me, and several of you have helped bring *Hormonious* to life. Thank you, Tracy, for your creative input and unending support, and Lauri, for helping me tweak my words for the better. Susan, you are simply a sparkling wordsmith superstar. Kathy and Ronda, your feedback was generous and welcome—thank you for taking the time. Thank you, my beloved sweet friends, for your unwavering friendship and love—Jeannie, Jodi, Julie, and Pam. You are my angels and I love you.

The online world is where I spend an enormous amount of time. Setting me on the right path began with Marie Forleo. You are a rockstar extraordinaire, and continue to inspire me every Tuesday. Selena Soo, you are on a mission and I'm fortunate to have entered your air space. Thank you for creating a spot in this world for introverts to thrive.

It apparently takes a village not only to write a book but to get it into the hands of others. Lari and Alex, you have been instrumental in gently managing me forward. Additional big appreciation goes to a few crucial players in this process—Gio, Michala, and Nicole.

And, last but in no way least, Eve. I simply could not have done this without your expert editor's eye, ideas, and know-how. Thank you. From the bottom of my heart.

# RESOURCES

- The Institute of Functional Medicine: https://www.ifm.org

- For a referral to a FDN-P, please email support@afdnp.com.

- Functional Timeline: https://p.widencdn.net/jlilgf/ IFM---Timeline_Clinical_v3

- Go to wellnessgirl.net/hormoniousplan to download:
    - Functional Timeline Plus (See Chapter 1)
    - Hormonious Habit Master List
    - Hormonious EveryDay Plan
    - BONUS Food Fundamentals List

- Perceived Stress Scale: https://bit.ly/2FAjHNP

- Social Readjustment: https://bit.ly/2T2Iopk

- Profile of Mood States (POMS): https://bit.ly/37aIFPa

- Please check out the following programs. Some of them offer discount codes.
    - Filtered water. Learn which water filter is best

for your needs with this online program created by Lara Adler, an environmental toxin expert—https://www.laraadler.com/pure/

o   Soaking and Fermenting. Learn the proper method for soaking and fermenting foods with Sarica Cernohous—http://funkykitchenfresh.com/program/

o   Fermented Foods. Learn how to make fermented vegetables at home in Summer Bock's free online workshop. After you register, you'll receive a 25% off coupon code to apply to her Fermented Foods 101 course. www.gutrebuilding.com/hormonious.

o   Dry Farm Wines (a bottle of wine for a penny): https://www.dryfarmwines.com/wellnessgirl

# EXPERTS

A few who have informed my knowledge and who can be a resource for you.

- Daniel Amen, MD

- Josh Axe, DNM, DC, CNS

- Kelly Brogan, MD

- Hyla Cass, MD

- Alan Christianson, ND

- Walter Crinnion, ND

- Felice Gersh, MD

- Trupti Gokani, MD

- Mark Hyman, MD

- Dan Kalish, DC

- Datis Kharrazian, DHSc, DC, MS

- Chris Kresser, M.S. L.Ac (Paleo)

- Ben Lynch, ND

- Deanna Minich, Ph.D.

- Amy Myers, MD

- Andrea Nakayama,

- Tom O'Bryan, DC, CCN, DACBN

- Vincent Pedre, MD

- David Perlmutter, MD

- Allison Siebecker, ND, MSOM, LAc (SIBO)

- Terry Wahls, MD

- Andrew Weil, MD

# ABOUT THE AUTHOR

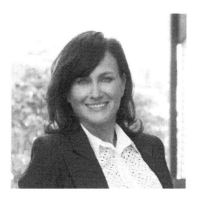

Karen Bernstein Shoshana, the founder and lead health expert at wellnessgirl.net, has helped her clients overcome chronic health issues including stress, fatigue, sleeplessness, resistant weight loss, and digestive challenges. A former attorney certified in Functional Diagnostic Nutrition, Karen uses her extensive education in functional medicine, nutrition, and holistic health counseling to get to the underlying cause(s) and guide her clients to whole body health.

The spark came from a crisis in 2006, when her mother was diagnosed with Alzheimer's Disease. Learning how to meditate as a way to cope and to support her mother, Karen was hit with a huge *a-ha* about the mind-body connection and the healing possibilities of meditation.

Beyond that, seeing her mother lose command of her own faculties inspired Karen to pivot from law to a career that would help women take back control of their bodies and health. Her signature mandate works—she inspires them to become the CEOs of their bodies.

Topics Karen specializes in and speaks on include digestive and hormonal health, nutrition, and lifestyle health. Karen has been a contributing writer to everydayHEALTH.com, featured as a health expert in Huffington Post, TEDx, and MakeItBetter.net, and is a member of the Institute for Functional Medicine.

Karen isn't just a grown-up wiz kid when it comes to the art and science of health. She's also keen on world travel, training her dog, and spending time in her favorite place, Michigan.

If you like this book, she welcomes your review on Amazon. Your honest feedback is sincerely appreciated.

Connect with her at any of the below:

http://fb.com/wellnessgirl

https://www.linkedin.com/in/wellnessgirl/

https://www.instagram.com/wellgirlwell/

# ENDNOTES

1    https://www.ifm.org

2    As a daughter of a physician, I was privy not only to trips to the hospital and my dad's office to visit his patients but also to box loads of antibiotics at the hint of a cough. That was the way things were done back then. At the first sign of a sore throat, I was instructed to a full course of those life-saving antibiotics, which, as you'll soon discover, is a likely contributing factor to some of the most vexing health issues.

3    NICHDPress. "NIH Study of WWII Evacuees Suggests Mental Illness May Be Passed to Offspring." *EurekAlert!*

4    Goosby, Bridget J., and Chelsea Heidbrink. *Advances in Pediatrics.*, U.S. National Library of Medicine, 1 Aug. 2013.

5    Yehuda, Rachel, et al. "Holocaust Exposure Induced Intergenerational Effects on FKBP5 Methylation." *Biological Psychiatry*, vol. 80, no. 5, 2016, pp. 372–380., doi:10.

6    https://www.ifm.org

7    If you'd like to know more about the toxins in your environment, this company produces a wearable band that measures them—http://www.myexposome.com.

8    An acronym for **F**ermentable **O**ligo-, **D**i-, **M**ono-saccharides **A**nd **P**olyols. FODMAPs are short-chain carbohydrates (sugars) that can be difficult to digest for some. A FODMAPs diet is often recommended for those who suffer from symptoms of IBS and SIBO.

9    Gut and Psychology Syndrome Diet created by Dr. Natasha Campbell McBride removes grains, starchy vegetables and refined carbs. It is a therapeutic intervention commonly used to treat ADD/ADHD, autism, dyspraxia, schizophrenia, depression, digestive disorders, food allergies, learning disabilities, and sensitivities and autoimmunity conditions.

10    http://wellnessgirl.net/rebootcleanse/

11    After much research, we found an ethical company that appeared to treat their elephants well.

12    H. pylori is typically found in the stomach. There is some controversy as to whether this bacteria poses a risk, as half the world's population has H. pylori with no symptoms. Consult an FM practitioner if H. pylori is a concern for you.

13    Among these functions are digestion, assimilation, nutrient distribution, tissue uptake and use of nutrients at specific cellular sites. Liska, DeAnn, and Jeffrey Bland. *Clinical Nutrition: a Functional Approach.* 2nd ed., Institute for FM, 2004.

14    The small intestines is comprised of the duodenum, in which most of our digestion takes place, the jejunum, where most of absorption takes place and the ilium, which absorbs Vitamin B12, bile salts and whatever products of digestion are not absorbed in the jejunum.

15    To cross the intestinal barrier, proteins need to be broken down into amino acids, fat into fatty acids, and carbs into glucose, fructose, or galactose.

16    Koh, H.; Lee, MJ.; Kim, MJ.; Shin, JL.; Chung, KS. (February 2010). "Simple diagnostic approach to childhood fecal retention using the Leech score and Bristol stool form scale in medical practice". *J Gastroenterol Hepatol.* 25 (2): 334–8.

17    Mueller, Noel T., et al. *Trends in Molecular Medicine*, U.S. National Library of Medicine, Feb. 2015

18    Rodgers B, Kirley K, Mounsey A. Prescribing an antibiotic? Pair it with probiotics. Ewigman B, ed. *The Journal of Family Practice.* 2013;62(3):148-150.

19    Neuman, H. et al. "Microbial endocrinology: The interplay between the microbiota and the endocrine system." FEMS Microbiol Rev. 2015 Jul;39(4):509-21.

20    Kwa, M, et al. "The Intestinal Microbiome and Estrogen Receptor-Positive Female Breast Cancer." *Advances in Pediatrics.*, U.S. National Library of Medicine, 22 Apr. 2016.

21    Li, Jau-Yi, et al. "Sex Steroid Deficiency–Associated Bone Loss Is Microbiota Dependent and Prevented by Probiotics." *The Journal of Clinical Investigation*, American Society for Clinical Investigation, 1 June 2016.

22    Baker, L, et al. "The Role of Estrogen in Cardiovascular Disease." *The Journal of Surgical Research.*, U.S. National Library of Medicine, Dec. 2003.

23    Lizcano, Fernando, and Guillermo Guzmán. "Estrogen Deficiency and the Origin of Obesity during Menopause." *BioMed Research International*, Hindawi Publishing Corporation, 2014.

24    Baker, J M, et al. "Estrogen-Gut Microbiome Axis: Physiological and Clinical Implications." *Maturitas.*, U.S. National Library of Medicine, Sept. 2017.

25    Utzeri, E., & Usai, P. (2017). "Role of non-steroidal anti-inflammatory drugs on intestinal permeability and nonalcoholic fatty liver disease." *World journal of gastroenterology, 23*(22), 3954–3963.

26    Leccioli, V., Oliveri, M., Romeo, M., Berretta, M., & Rossi, P. (2017). "A New Proposal for the Pathogenic Mechanism of Non-Coeliac/Non-Allergic Gluten/Wheat Sensitivity: Piecing Together the Puzzle of Recent Scientific Evidence." *Nutrients, 9*(11), 1203.

27    Fasano, Alessio. *Clinical Gastroenterology and Hepatology : the Official Clinical Practice Journal of the American Gastroenterological Association*, U.S. National Library of Medicine, Oct. 2012.

28    https://www.ifm.org

29    Ford, Alexander C. et al. "Small Intestinal Bacterial Overgrowth in Irritable Bowel Syndrome: Systematic Review and Meta-analysis." Clinical Gastroenterology and Hepatology, December 2009, Volume 7, Issue 12, 1279 – 1286.

30    Patil, Anant D. "Link Between Hypothyroidism and Small Intestinal Bacterial Overgrowth." *Indian Journal of Endocrinology and Metabolism*, Medknow Publications & Media Pvt Ltd, 2014.

31    Mercier, Paul, and Pierre Poitras. "Gastrointestinal Symptoms and Masticatory Dysfunction." *Journal of Gastroenterology and Hepatology*, vol. 7, no. 1, 1992, pp. 61–65.

32    Readfearn, Graham. "WHO Launches Health Review after Microplastics Found in 90% of Bottled Water." HuffPost, 16 Mar. 2018.

33    Environmental Working Group. "EWG's Tap Water Database: What's in Your Drinking Water?" https://www.ewg.org/tapwater/index.php#.Wu_4FS-ZNn6.

34    Everett ET. "Fluoride's Effects on the Formation of Teeth and Bones, and the Influence of Genetics." *Journal of Dental Research.* 2011;90(5):552-560. doi:10.1177/0022034510384626.

35    Spak CJ, Sjöstedt S, Eleborg L, Veress B, Perbeck L, Ekstrand J. "Tissue response of gastric mucosa after ingestion of fluoride." *BMJ : British Medical Journal.* 1989;298(6689):1686-1687.

36    Italian volcano brand is available in many markets.

37    http://wellnessgirl.net/rebootcleanse/

38    Gupta, Raj Kishor, Shivraj Singh Gangoliya, and Nand Kumar Singh. "Reduction of Phytic Acid and Enhancement of Bioavailable Micronutrients in Food Grains." *Journal of Food Science and Technology* 52.2 (2015): 676–684. *PMC*. Web. 7 May 2018.

39   Chavan, J K, and S Kadam. "Nutritional Improvement of Cereals by Sprouting." *Advances in Pediatrics.*, U.S. National Library of Medicine.

40   Chung, T Y, et al. "Compositional and Digestibility Changes in Sprouted Barley and Canola Seeds." *Advances in Pediatrics.*, U.S. National Library of Medicine, Sept. 1989.

41   Gupta, H O. "Protein Quality Evaluation of Sprouted Maize." *Plant Foods for Human Nutrition (Dordrecht, Netherlands).*, U.S. National Library of Medicine, July 1994.

42   Jeffery IB, Lynch DB, O'Toole PW. "Composition and temporal stability of the gut microbiota in older persons." ISME J. 2016;10(1):170–82.

43   Zapata HJ, Quagliarello VJ. "The Microbiota and Microbiome in Aging: Potential Implications in Health and Age-related Diseases." *Journal of the American Geriatrics Society.* 2015;63(4):776-781.

44   https://functionaldiagnosticnutrition.com

45   Liska, *Clinical Nutrition*, 205.

46   Rao, R., & Samak, G. (2012). "Role of Glutamine in Protection of Intestinal Epithelial Tight Junctions." *Journal of epithelial biology & pharmacology*, 5(Suppl 1-M7), 47–54.

47   Choi, Y. K., & Park, K. G. (2018). "Targeting Glutamine Metabolism for Cancer Treatment." *Biomolecules & therapeutics*, 26(1), 19–28.

48   https://functionaldiagnosticnutrition.com

49   Mysels, David J, and Maria A Sullivan. "The relationship between opioid and sugar intake: review of evidence and clinical applications." *Journal of opioid management* vol. 6,6 (2010): 445-52.

50   Ulrich-Lai, Yvonne M. et al. "Pleasurable Behaviors Reduce Stress via Brain Reward Pathways." *Proceedings of the National Academy of Sciences of the United States of America* 107.47 (2010): 20529–20534. *PMC*. Web. 7 May 2018.

51   "Grin and Bear It! Smiling Facilitates Stress Recovery." *Association for Psychological Science*, www.psychologicalscience.org/news/releases/smiling-facilitates-stress-recovery.html.

52   Lawrence, Elizabeth A., et al. "Happiness and Longevity in the United States." *Social Science & Medicine*, Volume 145, November 2015, Pages 115-119.

53   Goyal, Madhav, et al. "Meditation Programs for Psychological Stress and Well-Being." *JAMA Internal Medicine*, vol. 174, no. 3, Jan. 2014, p. 357.

54   Marchand, William R. "Mindfulness-Based Stress Reduction, Mindfulness-Based Cognitive Therapy, and Zen Meditation for Depression, Anxiety, Pain,

and Psychological Distress." *Journal of Psychiatric Practice*, vol. 18, no. 4, 2012, pp. 233–252.

55    Klepeis, Neil E, et al. "The National Human Activity Pattern Survey (NHAPS): a Resource for Assessing Exposure to Environmental Pollutants." *Journal of Exposure Science & Environmental Epidemiology*, vol. 11, no. 3, 2001, pp. 231–252.

56    Lee, Min-sun et al. "Interaction with Indoor Plants May Reduce Psychological and Physiological Stress by Suppressing Autonomic Nervous System Activity in Young Adults: A Randomized Crossover Study." *Journal of Physiological Anthropology* 34.1 (2015): 21. *PMC*. Web. 7 May 2018.

57    Richards, Louise M. "NASA Technical Reports Server (NTRS)2008364NASA Technical Reports Server (NTRS). Washington, DC. NASA Conter for Aerospace Information Last Visited June 2008. Gratis URL: Http://Ntrs.nasa. gov/." *Reference Reviews*, vol. 22, no. 8, 2008, pp. 40–41.

58    "Plants Clean Air and Water for Indoor Environments". Public Safety, Originating Technology/NASA contribution.https://spinoff.nasa.gov/ Spinoff2007/ps_3.html.

59    Nieuwenhuis, M, et al. "The Relative Benefits of Green versus Lean Office Space: Three Field Experiments." *Journal of Experimental Psychology. Applied.*, U.S. National Library of Medicine, Sept. 2014.

60    Hansen, Anita L. et al. "Fish Consumption, Sleep, Daily Functioning, and Heart Rate Variability." *Journal of Clinical Sleep Medicine : JCSM : Official Publication of the American Academy of Sleep Medicine* 10.5 (2014): 567–575. *PMC*. Web. 7 May 2018.

61    Kiecolt-Glaser, Janice K. et al. "Omega-3 Supplementation Lowers Inflammation and Anxiety in Medical Students: A Randomized Controlled Trial." *Brain, behavior, and immunity* 25.8 (2011): 1725-1734. *PMC*. Web. 7 May 2018.

62    Chandrasekhar, K., Jyoti Kapoor, and Sridhar Anishetty. "A Prospective, Randomized Double-Blind, Placebo-Controlled Study of Safety and Efficacy of a High-Concentration Full-Spectrum Extract of *Ashwagandha* Root in Reducing Stress and Anxiety in Adults." *Indian Journal of Psychological Medicine* 34.3 (2012): 255–262. *PMC*. Web. 7 May 2018.

63    Panossian, Alexander, and Georg Wikman. "Evidence-Based Efficacy of Adaptogens in Fatigue, and Molecular Mechanisms Related to Their Stress-Protective Activity." *Current Clinical Pharmacology*, vol. 4, no. 3, Jan. 2009, pp. 198–219.

64    Cohen, Marc Maurice. "Tulsi - *Ocimum Sanctum*: A Herb for All Reasons." *Journal of Ayurveda and Integrative Medicine* 5.4 (2014): 251–259. *PMC*. Web. 7 May 2018.

65    Peters, E. M., et al. "Vitamin C Supplementation Attenuates the Increases in Circulating Cortisol, Adrenaline and Anti-Inflammatory Polypeptides Following Ultramarathon Running." *International Journal of Sports Medicine*, vol. 22, no. 7, 2001, pp. 537–543.

66    Yeap, Swee Keong et al. "Antistress and Antioxidant Effects of Virgin Coconut Oil *in Vivo*." *Experimental and Therapeutic Medicine* 9.1 (2015): 39–42. *PMC*. Web. 7 May 2018.

67    Meissner, H. O. et al. "Hormone-Balancing Effect of Pre-Gelatinized Organic Maca (*Lepidium Peruvianum* Chacon): (I) Biochemical and Pharmacodynamic Study on Maca Using Clinical Laboratory Model on Ovariectomized Rats." *International Journal of Biomedical Science : IJBS* 2.3 (2006): 260–272.

68    Chen, Chun-Qiu et al. "Distribution, Function and Physiological Role of Melatonin in the Lower Gut." *World Journal of Gastroenterology : WJG* 17.34 (2011): 3888–3898. *PMC*. Web. 7 May 2018.

69    Burke, Tina M. et al. "Effects of Caffeine on the Human Circadian Clock *in Vivo* and *in Vitro*." *Science translational medicine* 7.305 (2015): 305ra146. *PMC*. Web. 7 May 2018.

70    Mortavazi, Seyed et al. "Alterations in TSH and Thyroid Hormones Following Mobile Phone Use." *Oman Medical Journal* 24.4 (2009): 274–278. *PMC*. Web. 7 May 2018.

71    De Coster, Sam, and Nicolas van Larebeke. "Endocrine-Disrupting Chemicals: Associated Disorders and Mechanisms of Action." *Journal of Environmental and Public Health* 2012 (2012): 713696. *PMC*. Web. 7 May 2018.

72    Perlmutter, David. *Grain Brain: the Surprising Truth about Wheat, Carbs, and Sugar—Your Brain's Silent Killers*. Little Brown, 2015.

73    Baron, Kelly Glazer, Kathryn J. Reid, and Phyllis C. Zee. "Exercise to Improve Sleep in Insomnia: Exploration of the Bidirectional Effects." *Journal of Clinical Sleep Medicine : JCSM : Official Publication of the American Academy of Sleep Medicine* 9.8 (2013): 819–824. *PMC*. Web. 7 May 2018.

74    "How Does Exercise Help Those with Chronic Insomnia?" *National Sleep Foundation*, sleepfoundation.org/ask-the-expert/ how-does-exercise-help-those-chronic-insomnia.

75    Cameron, Julia. *The Artist's Way: A Spiritual Path to Higher Creativity*. New York: J.P. Tarcher/ Putnam, 2002.

76    Kim, In-Hee et al. "Essential Oil Inhalation on Blood Pressure and Salivary Cortisol Levels in Prehypertensive and Hypertensive Subjects." *Evidence-based Complementary and Alternative Medicine : eCAM* 2012 (2012): 984203. *PMC*. Web. 7 May 2018.

77    Reiter, R.j. "Electromagnetic Fields and Melatonin Production." *Biomedicine & Pharmacotherapy*, vol. 47, no. 10, 1993, pp. 439–444.

78    Peuhkuri, Katri, Nora Sihvola, and Riitta Korpela. "Dietary Factors and Fluctuating Levels of Melatonin." *Food & Nutrition Research* 56 (2012): 10.3402/ fnr.v56i0.17252. *PMC*. Web. 7 May 2018.

79    Hansen, Anita L. et al. "Fish Consumption, Sleep, Daily Functioning, and Heart Rate Variability." *Journal of Clinical Sleep Medicine : JCSM : Official Publication of the American Academy of Sleep Medicine* 10.5 (2014): 567–575. *PMC*. Web. 7 May 2018.

80    Gominak, S.c., and W.e. Stumpf. "The World Epidemic of Sleep Disorders Is Linked to Vitamin D Deficiency." *Medical Hypotheses*, vol. 79, no. 2, 2012, pp. 132–135.

81    Crook T, Petrie W, Wells C, Massari DC., Effects of phosphatidylserine in Alzheimer's disease. Psychopharmacol Bull. 1992;28(1):61-6.

82    Hellhammer J, Vogt D, Franz N, Freitas U, Rutenberg D. "A soy-based phosphatidylserine/ phosphatidic acid complex (PAS) normalizes the stress reactivity of hypothalamus-pituitary-adrenal-axis in chronically stressed male subjects: a randomized, placebo-controlled study." Lipids Health Dis. 2014 Jul 31;13:121. doi: 10.1186/1476-511X-13-121.

83    Barth, Claudia, Arno Villringer, and Julia Sacher. "Sex Hormones Affect Neurotransmitters and Shape the Adult Female Brain during Hormonal Transition Periods." *Frontiers in Neuroscience* 9 (2015): 37. *PMC*. Web. 7 May 2018.

84    Parry, Barbara L. "Optimal Management of Perimenopausal Depression." *International Journal of Women's Health* 2 (2010): 143–151.

85    Rekkas, Paraskevi Vivien, et al. "Greater Monoamine Oxidase A Binding in Perimenopausal Age as Measured With Carbon 11–Labeled Harmine Positron Emission Tomography."*JAMA Psychiatry*, vol. 71, no. 8, Jan. 2014, p. 873.

86    "The Brain Gut Connection." Johns Hopkins Medicine, www.hopkinsmedicine. org/health/ healthy_aging/healthy_body/the-brain-gut-connection.

87    Liska, *Clinical Nutrition.*

88    Rao, T.S. Sathyanarayana et al.  "Understanding Nutrition, Depression and Mental Illnesses."  *Indian Journal of Psychiatry* 50.2 (2008): 77-82. PMC. Web. 7 May 2018.

89    de Oliveira I J, et al. "Effects of Oral Vitamin C Supplementation on Anxiety in Students: A Double-Blind, Randomized, Placebo-controlled Trial." *Pakistan Journal of Biological Sciences: PJBS.*, U.S. National Library of Medicine, Jan. 2015.

90    Kossman, D A, et al. "Exercise Lowers Estrogen and Progesterone Levels in Premenopausal Women at High Risk of Breast Cancer." *Journal of Applied Physiology* (Bethesda, Md.: 1985.

91    Tremblay, A, et al. "Impact of Exercise Intensity on Body Fatness and Skeletal Muscle Metabolism." *Metabolism: Clinical and Experimental.*, U.S. National Library of Medicine, July 1994.

92    Words of Senator Kamala Harris.

93    Clapp, Megan, et al. "Gut Microbiota's Effect on Mental Health: the Gut-Brain Axis." *Clinics and Practice*, vol. 7, no. 4, 2017.

94    Liska, *Clinical Nutrition.*

95    Shimizu, Kuniyoshi, et al. "Reduction of Depression and Anxiety by 4 Weeks Hericium Erinaceus Intake." *Plant Production Science*, Crop Science Society of Japan, 8 Sept. 2010.

96    Wong, Kah-Hui, et al. "Neuroregenerative Potential of Lion's Mane Mushroom, Hericium Erinaceus (Bull.: Fr.) Pers. (Higher Basidiomycetes), in the Treatment of Peripheral Nerve Injury (Review)." *International Journal of Medicinal Mushrooms*, vol. 14, no. 5, 2012, pp. 427–446., doi:10.

97    Adapted from Dr. Frank Lipman.

98    Bravo, J. A., et al. "Ingestion of Lactobacillus Strain Regulates Emotional Behavior and Central GABA Receptor Expression in a Mouse via the Vagus Nerve." *Proceedings of the National Academy of Sciences*, vol. 108, no. 38, 2011, pp. 16050–16055.

99    Peterson, Christine Tara, Kate Denniston, and Deepak Chopra. "Therapeutic Uses of *Triphala* in Ayurvedic Medicine." *Journal of Alternative and Complementary Medicine* 23.8 (2017): 607–614. PMC. Web. 7 May 2018.

100   Kamali, Seyed Hamid et al. "Efficacy of 'Itrifal Saghir', a Combination of Three Medicinal Plants in the Treatment of Obesity; A Randomized Controlled Trial." *DARU Journal of Pharmaceutical Sciences* 20.1 (2012): 33. PMC. Web. 7 May 2018.

101   Blessing, E M, et al. "Cannabidiol as a Potential Treatment for Anxiety Disorders." *Neurotherapeutics : the Journal of the American Society for Experimental NeuroTherapeutics.*, U.S. National Library of Medicine, Oct. 2015.

102   Babson, K A, et al. "Cannabis, Cannabinoids, and Sleep: a Review of the Literature." *Current Psychiatry Reports.*, U.S. National Library of Medicine, Apr. 2017.

103   Booth, Frank W., Christian K. Roberts, and Matthew J. Laye. "Lack of Exercise Is a Major Cause of Chronic Diseases." *Comprehensive Physiology* 2.2 (2012): 1143–1211. PMC. Web. 7 May 2018.

104 Tabish, Syed Amin. "Is Diabetes Becoming the Biggest Epidemic of the Twenty-First Century?" *International Journal of Health Sciences* 1.2 (2007): V–VIII. Print.

105 Denny-Brown, S., et al. "The Association of Macro- and Micronutrient Intake with Growth Hormone Secretion." *Growth Hormone & IGF Research*, vol. 22, no. 3-4, 2012, pp. 102–107.

106 Prinz, Patricia N., et al. "Effect of Alcohol on Sleep and Nighttime Plasma Growth Hormone and Cortisol Concentrations." *The Journal of Clinical Endocrinology & Metabolism*, vol. 51, no. 4, 1980, pp. 759–764.

107 Mattson MP, Wan R. "Beneficial effects of intermittent fasting and caloric restriction on the cardiovascular and cerebrovascular systems." *J Nutr Biochem.* 2005 Mar;16(3):129-37.

108 Collier R. (2013). "Intermittent fasting: the science of going without." *CMAJ : Canadian Medical Association journal = journal de l'Association medicale canadienne*, 185(9), E363–E364.

109 Wei, Min, et al. "Fasting-Mimicking Diet and Markers/Risk Factors for Aging, Diabetes, Cancer, and Cardiovascular Disease." Science Translational Medicine, American Association for the Advancement of Science, 15 Feb. 2017, stm.sciencemag.org/content/9/377/eaai8700.

110 University of Surrey. (2018, August 30). "Changes in breakfast and dinner timings can reduce body fat." *ScienceDaily.*

111 "Endocrine Disruptors." *National Institute of Environmental Health Sciences*, U.S. Department of Health and Human Services.

112 Duty, S M, et al. "The Relationship between Environmental Exposures to Phthalates and DNA Damage in Human Sperm Using the Neutral Comet Assay." *Environmental Health Perspectives.*

113 Pekcici, Recep, et al. "Effects of Lead on Thyroid Functions in Lead-Exposed Workers." *SpringerLink*, Springer, Dordrecht, 12 Sept. 2009.

114 Godfrey, R J, et al. "The Exercise-Induced Growth Hormone Response in Athletes." *Sports Medicine* (Auckland, N.Z.).

115 Welbourne, T C. "Increased Plasma Bicarbonate and Growth Hormone after an Oral Glutamine Load." *The American Journal of Clinical Nutrition.*, U.S. National Library of Medicine, May 1995.

116 Berk, LS. "Studying the biology of hope: An interview with Lee S. Berk, DrPH, MPH. Interview by Sheldon Lewis." Adv Mind Body Med. 2007 Summer;22(2):28-31.

117 Nadeem, Maria. "Mindful Eating Verses Mindless Eating." *Advances in Obesity, Weight Management & Control*, vol. 4, no. 3, 2016.

118  "Dining out Associated with Increased Exposure to Harmful Chemicals Called Phthalates." *EurekAlert!*, eurekalert.org/pub_releases/2018-03/gwu-doa032318.php.

119  Kanaley JA. "Growth hormone, arginine and exercise." Curr Opin Clin Nutr Metab Care. 2008 Jan;11(1):50-4.

120  http://wellnessgirl.net/freedownload/

121  Avena, N. M., Rada, P., & Hoebel, B. G. (2008). Evidence for sugar addiction: behavioral and neurochemical effects of intermittent, excessive sugar intake. *Neuroscience and biobehavioral reviews, 32*(1), 20–39. https://doi.org/10.1016/j.neubiorev.2007.04.019

122  Cock, Peter De, and Claire-Lise Bechert. "Erythritol. Functionality in Noncaloric Functional Beverages." *Pure and Applied Chemistry*, vol. 74, no. 7, Jan. 2002, pp. 1281–1289.

123  Erythritol does not contain ethanol and is unrelated to alcoholic beverages.

124  Storey, D, et al. "Gastrointestinal Tolerance of Erythritol and Xylitol Ingested in a Liquid." *European Journal of Clinical Nutrition.*, U.S. National Library of Medicine, Mar. 2007.

125  Leidy HJ, et al. "The role of protein in weight loss and maintenance." Am J Clin Nutr. 2015 Apr 29.

126  Liska, *Clinical Nutrition.*

127  St-Onge, M P, and Bosarge, A. "Weight-Loss Diet That Includes Consumption of Medium- Chain Triacylglycerol Oil Leads to a Greater Rate of Weight and Fat Mass Loss than Does Olive Oil." *The American Journal of Clinical Nutrition.*, U.S. National Library of Medicine, Mar. 2008.

128  Liska, *Clinical Nutrition.*

129  Visit https://www.ifm.org or Resources for options.

130  nanograms per milliliter

131  http://wellnessgirl.net/recipe/go-to-salad/

Made in the USA
Columbia, SC
01 July 2022

62634600R00171